about this handbook

- This book is for you if you care for someone in the middle to late stages of dementia.

- Every person with dementia is different.

- Dementia can bring many problems, but not all of them will happen to any one person.

- When you read through this book, remember that the person you care for will not experience everything you read about.

- This book is designed to help you cope, not to worry you!

This book contains information and advice for people who care for someone in the middle to late stages of dementia (moderate to severe dementia). It aims to:

- help you feel less alone

- give you practical advice on coping

- help you to find caring more rewarding and less stressful

- show you where to go for help and for more information.

If you are supporting someone with mild dementia, or have a recent diagnosis yourself, you should read *Facing dementia* and *Don't make the journey alone* instead. They are both available free from the Dementia Helpline.

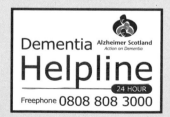

If you want to talk about anything you have read, or would like more information or local contacts, you can call the 24-hour Dementia Helpline. The number is **0808 808 3000** and all calls are free.

Note: As more women than men have dementia, we decided to call the person with dementia 'she' in this book. Using 'he or she' all the time can be awkward to read. However, the information applies just as much to men who have dementia.

contents

about dementia

coping with caring

money and legal matters

practical caring

long-stay care

further information

index

about dementia

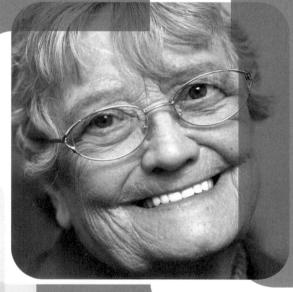
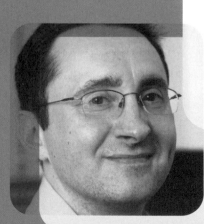

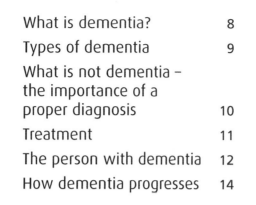

about dementia

What is dementia?

at a glance

- Dementia is an illness of the brain.
- The person with dementia will gradually start to need more and more help.
- Dementia affects older people most often.
- More rarely, people in their 40s or 50s or younger can get dementia.

Dementia is an illness of the brain. When someone has dementia, brain cells are damaged and die faster than they do normally. Losing brain cells means that the person's brain does not work as well as it should. Gradually the person begins to lose the ability to do things. Often it affects memory first. The person may become confused about where she is, what day it is and who people are. Everyday tasks become more and more difficult. Her personality may change.

Dementia is progressive, and the person will get gradually less and less able. However, this usually happens very slowly. Little by little, the person will need more help. Eventually someone with dementia will be unable to manage even basic tasks like eating, dressing and going to the toilet. But this will not happen suddenly. The illness can last many years.

At present there is no cure for dementia. But there is a lot you can do. This book is about how you can help.

Dementia affects about 2% of people aged 65 to 70, 5% of people aged 70 to 80 and about 20% over 80. Because people are living longer now, there are more people with dementia. It can also affect people in their 40s or 50s or even younger, although this is rarer. This is called early-onset dementia because it affects people at a relatively young age.

Types of dementia

at a glance

- There are many diseases which can cause dementia.
- Alzheimer's disease is the best known.
- Different kinds of dementia can lead to different problems, and each person is different.
- Not every problem will happen to the person you care for.

There are many diseases which can cause dementia. The best known is **Alzheimer's disease**. Alzheimer's disease probably causes more than half of all cases of dementia. When someone has Alzheimer's disease, individual brain cells are damaged. Gradually more and more brain cells fail to work properly. The result is a slow decline of mental powers.

Second most common is **vascular dementia**, including **multi-infarct dementia**. In these types of dementia, the blood supply to the brain is damaged in some way. In multi-infarct dementia, tiny 'strokes' (called infarcts) cut off the blood supply to small areas of the brain and the brain cells die. These strokes may be so small that no one notices them at the time. But the person may get worse quite suddenly, and then not change until the next stroke. So the progression of the illness can happen in a step-like way. It is often quite difficult for doctors to tell the difference between Alzheimer's disease and vascular dementia and some people seem to have a mixture.

Lewy body dementia seems to be connected with Parkinson's disease. Some people with Parkinson's disease develop a form of dementia, but people with Lewy body dementia don't necessarily get symptoms of Parkinson's. People with this kind of dementia may be more likely to have hallucinations (seeing things that aren't there) or spells of distressed or disturbed behaviour. They can also be very sensitive to drugs which are sometimes used to help behaviour problems.

In **alcohol-related dementia** (which includes **Korsakoff's syndrome**), there are problems particularly with recent memory. It is caused by lack of vitamin B1, which is needed for the brain. Heavy drinkers may not be able to use the vitamin properly, and often don't eat well. People with alcohol-related dementia should not drink alcohol, as this will make their dementia get worse. In some alcohol-related dementia, the progression of the illness will stop if the person stops drinking.

Frontal lobe dementia (which includes Pick's disease) damages the part of the brain which helps you plan and check what you are doing. The person may be more likely to do things at the wrong time or in the wrong place, which can be embarrassing for the carer. Memory loss is not as common in this kind of dementia.

Other kinds of dementia include **AIDS-related dementia** and **Creutzfeld–Jacob disease**. Some people with Down's syndrome also develop dementia, often in middle age.

Carers sometimes think that the illness started with a crisis such as the death of a partner or moving house. These events do not themselves cause dementia, but they may make someone in the early stages more confused. She may find a new house very confusing, or her late partner may have been helping so much that no one else noticed a problem.

Different kinds of dementia can lead to different kinds of problem, and each person with dementia is different. It is impossible to know exactly which problems the person you care for will face. This book looks at how to cope with many of the difficulties dementia can cause. But remember, not all of them will happen to the person you care for.

If you would like to know more about dementia, ask the person's doctor and see the **Further information** section on pages 102–111.

What is not dementia – the importance of a proper diagnosis

at a glance

- Not everyone will get dementia in old age.
- Many things can cause forgetfulness or confusion, not just dementia.
- A proper diagnosis is very important.

Old age does not cause dementia. It is more common in very old people, but eighty per cent of people over 80 stay mentally alert. Most of us will become a little forgetful from time to time. This is quite normal.

If you know someone who is forgetful or confused, don't just assume it

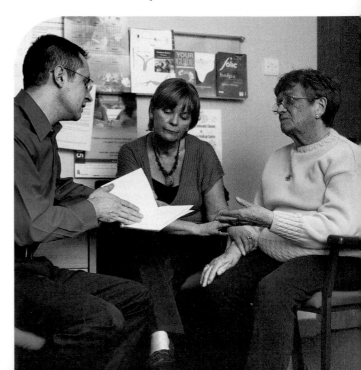

is dementia or 'just old age'. Try to persuade her to see a doctor. Memory loss and confusion are not always a sign of dementia. They can have a number of other causes. These include:

- infections, such as chest or urinary tract infections

- medicines, such as sleeping pills. If the dose is wrong or if the person takes several medicines together, this can lead to symptoms just like those of dementia

- various medical conditions such as heart or thyroid trouble

- stress, anxiety or depression.

These problems can all be successfully helped. The person's memory and mental function should then get back to normal.

It can be hard to make a firm diagnosis in the early stages. But if the doctor finds no other reason for the person's symptoms, he or she may diagnose dementia. It can be difficult to get the right help and advice until the person has a diagnosis.

Diagnosing what kind of dementia the person has is very important because it affects what treatment may be suitable.

The person's family doctor may refer her to a specialist for a diagnosis. Sometimes the family doctor may make the diagnosis. If you are not happy with the diagnosis, ask the doctor to refer the person to a specialist or to a memory clinic for a second opinion. The booklet *Getting help from your doctor* gives useful information – **call the Dementia Helpline on 0808 808 3000 for a free copy.**

Treatment
at a glance

- There are drug treatments which can help some people for a while.

- The drugs treat the symptoms – they are not cures.

- Other therapies may help the person deal with the effects of the illness.

- Ask the doctor about treatments or call the Dementia Helpline on 0808 808 3000 for more information.

Drug treatments are now available which can help some people. These drugs are not cures. They do not affect the underlying disease, and only help some people who try them.

For people with mild to moderate Alzheimer's disease or with Lewy body dementia, the treatments currently available are Aricept (donepezil), Exelon (rivastigmine) and Reminyl (galantamine). These are normally prescribed by hospital specialists, although in some areas general practitioners (GPs) may prescribe them. They all help brain cells pass messages between each other so that the person's brain can work a bit better. But they don't work for everyone, and they can have side effects.

A drug called Ebixa (memantine) can sometimes help people with moderate to severe Alzheimer's disease. It may also help in vascular dementia. However, it is not currently widely available on the NHS.

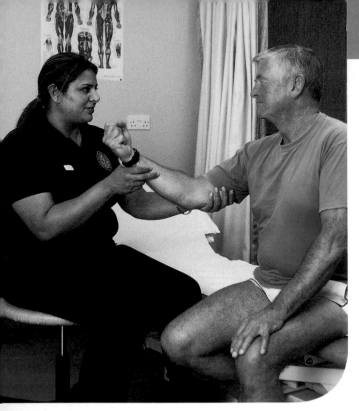

The person with dementia

at a glance

- Many people are now diagnosed early in the illness.
- The person with dementia will probably need emotional as well as practical support.
- Try to make sure that the person is as involved as possible in making decisions and choices.
- Remember the person with dementia's feelings and rights.

As well as drug treatment, there are other therapies which may help the person to deal with the effects of the illness. Ask the doctor about these. For example:

- speech and language therapy can help with communication or swallowing difficulties
- physiotherapy can help with mobility, reduce the risk of falls and help the person stay active
- a psychologist can help the person cope with difficulties including memory problems, behaviour changes or depression
- counselling can help in coming to terms with the illness.

Ask the doctor whether these treatments are appropriate. Call the Dementia Helpline for more information about treatments.

These days, many people are being diagnosed with dementia quite early on in the illness. This means that they are still able to take in the diagnosis and what it means for them. The person with dementia will probably need a lot of support, emotional as well as practical. Talk to the doctor or another health or social work professional about this. Perhaps the person could see a counsellor to help her cope.

For people in the early stages, the booklets *Facing dementia* and *Don't make the journey alone* (see **Further information,** pages 107–109) may be helpful. They are for people who have a diagnosis of dementia. It may help if someone reads the information together with the person, to help explain it.

Try to make sure that the person is as involved as possible in making decisions and choices about things that affect her (see **Money and legal matters**, page 28).

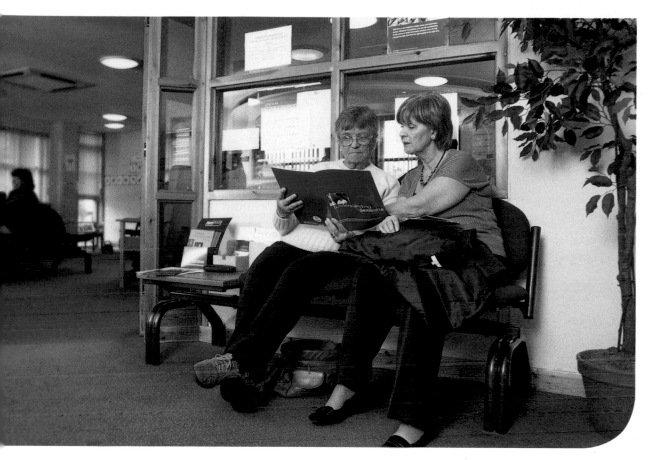

Remember that later on in the illness the person still has feelings, even if it may become more difficult to understand what she feels. She may be feeling depressed, frightened, frustrated or distressed. Try to work out what she is trying to communicate about her feelings. Be reassuring.

Enjoyable activities are important too. Although someone in the later stages of the illness may not remember an enjoyable event, she may still feel good during it and afterwards. It might be as simple as a piece of familiar music, a smile or a hug.

Don't be tempted to treat the person with dementia like a child. Even if she finds it hard to understand things, she is still an adult. She has a whole lifetime of experiences behind her, and an adult's needs, desires and rights.

How dementia progresses

at a glance

- The progress of dementia varies between different people.
- Early on the person may become forgetful or behave unusually.
- The person may realise something is wrong, and different people react to this differently.
- Later on the person will have more difficulties.
- The person you care for probably won't have all the problems in this book.
- The person will gradually need more and more help.
- Some of the difficulties you faced earlier on may no longer be a problem later in the illness.
- There are many ways of making life easier and happier for both the person with dementia and yourself.

The progress of the illness varies a lot from one person to another. This means that no one can give firm answers about what you can expect. The problems can also vary from day to day or even hour to hour. Some difficulties are more common early in the illness and others tend to happen later, but this too is variable. The illness may last many years, sometimes progressing faster, sometimes more slowly.

At first, the changes are slight. The person with dementia may become forgetful and likely to repeat things. She may behave in ways which are a bit odd for her.

She may understand that she has dementia and what this means for her, or she may realise that something is wrong but not fully grasp what it is. So she may be anxious, frightened that she is losing control or embarrassed by the mistakes she makes. Some people withdraw into themselves or become depressed. Some people lose interest and enthusiasm for things. Others seem to be less interested in their personal appearance or hygiene.

One man with dementia described feeling as though a fog was covering his mind, making it hard to think clearly. Sometimes, on better days, the fog would lift, and some days it would get thicker.

As the illness goes on, the changes are greater. Memory problems get worse. The person's behaviour may change too, and sometimes may be hard to understand or cope with. The person may:

- confuse the time of day, where she is or who people are
- lose things around the house
- get lost in previously familiar places
- not recognise everyday objects or what they are for
- not recognise friends or family
- get worse at practical skills, such as cooking or driving

- have difficulty managing or understanding money

- have difficulty making decisions about finances, property, welfare and health matters

- have difficulty in expressing herself when talking or writing (as she loses track of what she is saying or can't find the right words)

- find it hard to grasp what people say or things that are written

- repeat questions over and over again

- neglect personal care or home care

- need help with everyday tasks such as bathing and dressing

- not eat properly or overeat

- be up and about at night

- blame others for things she forgets she has done, or have other mistaken ideas

- become angry or upset very quickly or behave in other uncharacteristic ways

- have continence problems

- see or hear things that are not there (hallucinations).

These are all things which can go wrong when someone has dementia. But the person you care for probably won't have all these problems.

Because of these problems the person will gradually need more and more help.

Some of the difficulties you may have faced earlier on will no longer be a problem later in the illness.

For example, if the person was frustrated and aggressive, she will probably be calmer.

As time goes on, the person's whole personality may change a great deal. Some carers say that the person seems to have become 'a shadow of her former self'. But most people keep fairly strong physically for a long time. In the later stages of the illness, people with dementia become physically very frail. In the very last stages even the person's ability to resist simple infections is lost and, sadly, the illness is eventually fatal. But of course, because it is such a long-lasting illness, and because many people are older when they get it, many people with dementia die of completely unconnected causes.

Having read this far you may be feeling very anxious about the future. Looking after a person with dementia can be very hard, and it is understandable that many people find it a difficult or even impossible task. But others find the experience brings out unexpected inner strengths and that caring has its own rewards.

There are many ways of making life easier and happier for both the person with dementia and yourself. This book draws on the experience of carers and we hope that the ideas will help you.

15

coping with caring

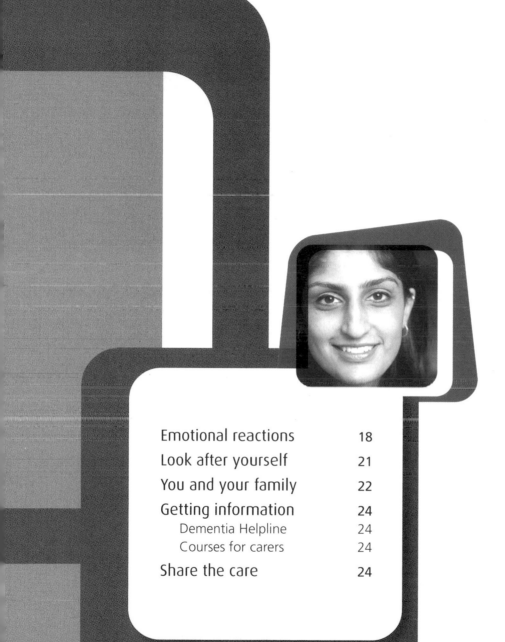

Emotional reactions

at a glance

- Caring can be both rewarding and stressful.
- Many things can affect your reactions.
- Talk about your feelings.
- Call the 24-hour Dementia Helpline free on **0808 808 3000** if you need to talk to someone.
- Join a carers' support group.
- Don't hide the fact that a relative has dementia.
- Don't assume that only the person you care for has a particular problem.
- Don't be too hard on yourself.

Looking after someone who has dementia can be very stressful. One of the things you may find hardest is living with your feelings about caring. It helps to know what these feelings might be.

Most carers experience a variety of emotions. The most common are sadness, guilt, anger and fear. Tiredness and tension are also common. Some of these feelings come as no surprise. You might expect to be sad when you feel you are slowly losing someone you love. Anger can be more of a shock. You may be alarmed at how frustrated and angry you can get. You may find you come to the end of your tether even over quite minor upsets.

On the other hand, caring can also be rewarding. For example, some people see it as a chance to give back to a parent the care they were given as a child. People with dementia often seem calm and happy despite the illness.

For many carers, there will be both rewarding and stressful times.

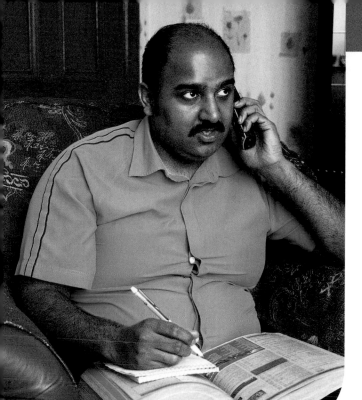

- **Particular problems that affect the person you are caring for.**
  For instance, night-time disturbance or constant demands for attention can be very stressful.

- **Changes in your lifestyle.**
  You may have given up a job or moved home to care for someone. You may be managing on less money than you used to have. You may feel isolated.

- **How much support you have.**
  Do you feel you are the only one looking after the person, or do other people share the care or share the responsibilities?

Other people may not see the changes in the person in the way that you do, as the carer. You know what effect the illness is having on her, but other people who aren't so close to her may only see her putting a good face on things. This can sometimes make it hard for people to understand what caring is really like for you.

Caring for someone you don't live with brings its own worries too. Many people who care at a distance worry a lot about safety. Some people feel guilty about not being there all the time. Some feel frustrated because they find it hard to know what is going on.

It is useful to work out what makes you feel most upset. This will help you to be clear about the kind of help you need to keep up the care. Start by talking about the problems you are facing and your feelings. Look after yourself and share the job of caring.

Many things can affect your reactions. For instance:

- **Your relationship with the person with dementia.**
  Someone you depended upon in the past may now be dependent on you. Or there may have been problems in your relationship in the past. Perhaps you are caring for your partner, and so no longer have the support you used to have in your relationship. You may miss things that kept you close, such as sharing problems and talking things out, or a sexual relationship.

- **Your reasons for caring.**
  People may find themselves looking after a relative because they want to, or from a sense of duty. Some may feel they have little choice, which can add to the strain.

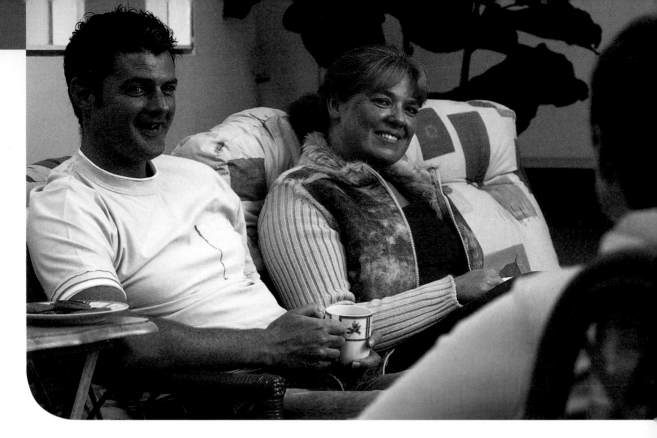

What you can do

1. It helps if you talk about your feelings rather than bottle them up. You may want to do this with a friend or member of your family, or you may want to talk to a professional such as a social worker or community psychiatric nurse, or both at different times.

2. The 24-hour Dementia Helpline is always there on **freephone 0808 808 3000.** Trained volunteers offer emotional support and information, whenever you want to call.

> *At the beginning just after my husband was diagnosed I found things very hard. But I got through it. I used to tell myself, 'I can cope for today and that's all I need for today. Tomorrow can look after itself.'*

3. In most areas there are carers' support groups. Talking to others in the same situation can be a great help. Even if there is no support group nearby, it is still worth trying to meet with someone else who looks after someone with dementia. Other carers, more than anyone else, can understand what you are going through. Ask the Dementia Helpline, community psychiatric nurse or the social work department about groups in your area.

4. Don't assume that only the person you care for has a particular problem. Other carers have probably been through the same kind of thing.

5. Some carers try to hide the fact that a relative has dementia. But dementia is an illness. It is not something to be ashamed of. It is not your fault, or your relative's. So try not to hide problems away or 'bottle them up'.

20

6. Practise saying the right things to yourself. Research has shown that how you react to a problem – what you tell yourself – affects the way you feel. So learn the habit of telling yourself things that help you feel good. If the long term looks bleak take one day at a time.

7. Try not to give yourself negative messages like, 'If anything else happens I'll never manage', or 'This is the last straw'. A more helpful approach is, 'I might not be doing a perfect job but I am doing quite well'. You may find it more important to remind yourself of these things when you are feeling low. Changing the things you say to yourself can have an amazing effect on how you feel.

> *When something goes wrong I say to myself, 'Relax, don't panic. I have coped so far and there is no reason why I won't continue to.' It seems to help, somehow.*

8. Don't be too hard on yourself. No one is perfect. It is normal to lose your patience sometimes. If you lose your temper and shout at or hit the person, talk to someone right away. The Dementia Helpline can help you decide what to do to get help so that it doesn't happen again. Calls are confidential and you don't have to give your name.

Look after yourself

at a glance

- Give yourself a break.
- Explain the situation to friends and family.
- Take time for yourself every day.
- Remember, looking after yourself is not selfish – it's sensible.

Sometimes carers feel as though they are being selfish if they take time for themselves or do some of the things they like to do. If you feel like that, ask yourself what you would say to someone else in your position.

> *My father used to follow me absolutely everywhere and I never had a moment to myself. I took to locking myself in the bathroom for half an hour when things got too much. I took a book with me and put my headphones on and just left him to it.*

Looking after yourself is not selfish – it's sensible. You need to look after yourself, physically and emotionally, if you want to be able to go on caring.

What you can do

1. Arrange for regular breaks to make sure you have time off. Family, friends, a local home support service and day centres can help (see page 77).

2. Try not to become isolated from friends and family. This often happens if the person with dementia behaves in an embarrassing way or you can't leave her on her own. Explain the situation to friends and tell them that you do want them to visit. Most will be glad to help and will soon get used to any unusual behaviour. The booklet *I'll get by with a little help from my friends* will help you explain to them what they can do to stay involved. Call the Dementia Helpline for a free copy.

3. Ask for respite breaks to give you a weekend, a week or more away from taking care of the person with dementia. This gives you the chance to recharge your batteries.

4. Take time for yourself. Think about what you find relaxing. For example, it might be listening to music, watching television, going for a walk, seeing friends or something else. Try to make sure you get some time each day to relax, even if it's only a few minutes.

5. Read Alzheimer Scotland's booklet *Looking after yourself* for more information on how carers can take care of themselves, and why they should. Call the Dementia Helpline for a free copy.

You and your family

at a glance

- **Talk to the whole family about the illness.**
- **Try to arrange some times when children can bring their friends home.**
- **Try not to let caring take over family life completely.**

For many carers, looking after someone with dementia brings changes in family relationships. Perhaps you have children who are also having to cope with the person's illness. But the time you spend caring can mean less time looking after them. Perhaps your children feel embarrassed to bring their friends to the house.

> *My husband is sometimes very good with our grandchildren, but sometimes he gets angry and they don't see why. The older ones understand a bit, but the youngest is only three and gets upset. I don't leave him alone with her any more.*
>
> *But I make sure they get times together doing something they enjoy and then I take her away again before he gets frustrated.*

They may worry about what the person might do. Perhaps you feel you are doing more than some other family members and resent that. Or maybe the rest of the family worry about you wearing yourself out.

There may be no simple solution. But there are some ideas which may help.

What you can do

1. Many people with dementia enjoy spending time with children and the children enjoy it too. Talk to children or grandchildren about the illness. Try to explain that any odd behaviour is not the person's fault. It is because she is ill. Offer to explain this to their friends too. The booklet *Understanding dementia – a guide for young carers* may help older children to understand – call the Dementia Helpline for a free copy.

2. Try to arrange some times when the person with dementia is out of the house so that children feel more able to bring their friends home. Perhaps she could go out with a friend or a home support worker sometimes. Try not to let caring take over family life completely. Ask for help to give you time off to spend with your family (see **Getting help** on page 76).

3. Talk to the rest of the family. Relatives not involved in day-to-day caring may not realise the demands on you. They may not understand the illness. Perhaps you could have a family discussion about how to care for the person with dementia.

4. If there are disagreements on what is best, it may help to ask someone else to take part in discussions, to make sure everyone gets a fair hearing. Perhaps a close friend, social worker, minister or the doctor could help.

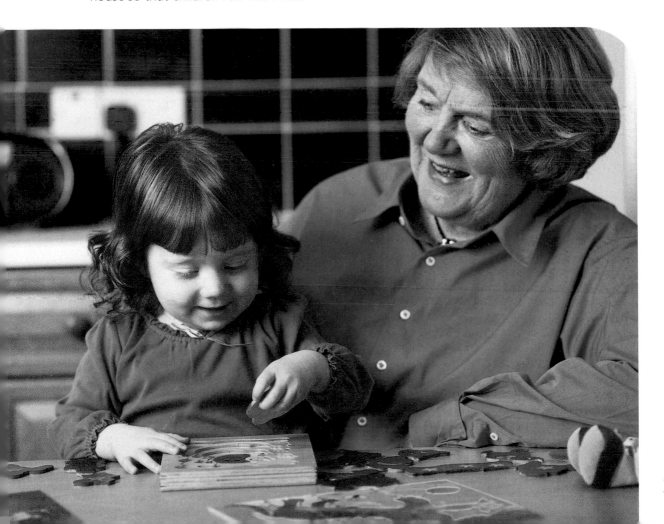

Getting information

at a glance

- Better information makes caring easier.
- Call the Dementia Helpline on 0808 808 3000.
- Go on a course for carers.

I was at a meeting with various professionals talking about my wife's dementia and they all seemed to talk in initials! 'CPN' this and 'OT' that. Finally I just told them that if they wanted to get any sense out of me they'd have to speak English. They all looked very embarrassed and apologised for using jargon.

It is easier to deal with caring when you have enough information. You may need information on the illness itself and how it will affect the person. You may need to find out about local services. Or you may want extra help with a particular problem.

Dementia Helpline

The 24-hour Dementia Helpline on **freephone 0808 808 3000** can provide information on almost anything. If the person who takes your call can't answer a question, he or she will try to find out. The Dementia Helpline is run by Alzheimer Scotland and has a panel of expert advisers.

Courses for carers

Although caring can be a full-time job, few carers get any training in how to do it. So you may feel you have to learn by trial and error. Alzheimer Scotland and carers' organisations arrange courses for carers through their local services. A carers' course can give you the chance to get accurate information about the illness, services available, financial and legal matters and how to cope. Research has shown that carers with this sort of training may feel less stressed than other carers. Call the Dementia Helpline to find out about a contact near you.

Share the care

at a glance

- Try to share caring with other members of the family and friends.
- Involve the person in discussions about her care as much as you can.
- Ask about what services are available.
- If you can no longer care for the person at home, discuss options with other members of the family and professionals.

Looking after someone with dementia can be a round-the-clock job. No one can provide all of the care, all of the time. Don't feel bad about accepting help. The help you need will change as time goes on. Get help as early on as possible. You may not feel you need much help now. But the person may find it easier

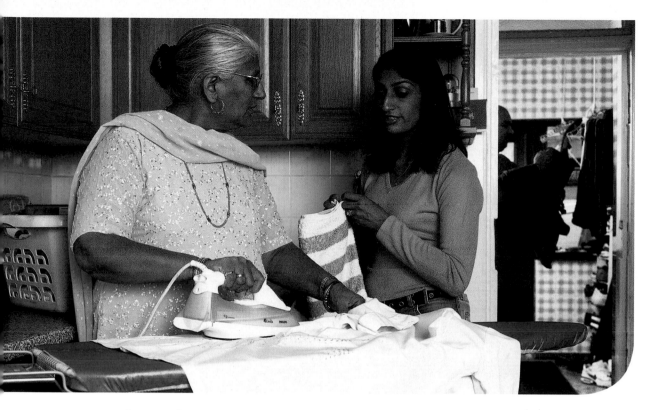

to get to know a home support worker, for example, earlier on in the illness.

What you can do

1. If possible, involve the person with dementia in discussions about her care. Try to make sure her wishes are heard.

2. If you can, try to share caring with other members of the family and friends.

3. Often people don't get help because no one realises they need it. So it is important to ask. Family, friends and neighbours may be more willing to help than you expect once you explain things to them.

4. Regular help with shopping, housework and caring for the person with dementia will allow you time for yourself. The person with dementia will enjoy having different company too.

5. Ask the social work department, community psychiatric nurse or doctor about what services are available. Ask the social work department for a community care assessment and a carer's assessment (see **Getting help**, page 76). It is important for both you and the person with dementia that you make full use of these services

6. There may come a time when it is no longer possible to care for the person with dementia at home. She may need to move into a care home or, in some cases, hospital care. It can be hard to decide when this time has come. You may find it easier to decide if you discuss it with other members of the family or professionals. If the person goes into a care home or hospital, you can still help care for her if you want to (see **Long-stay care**, page 92).

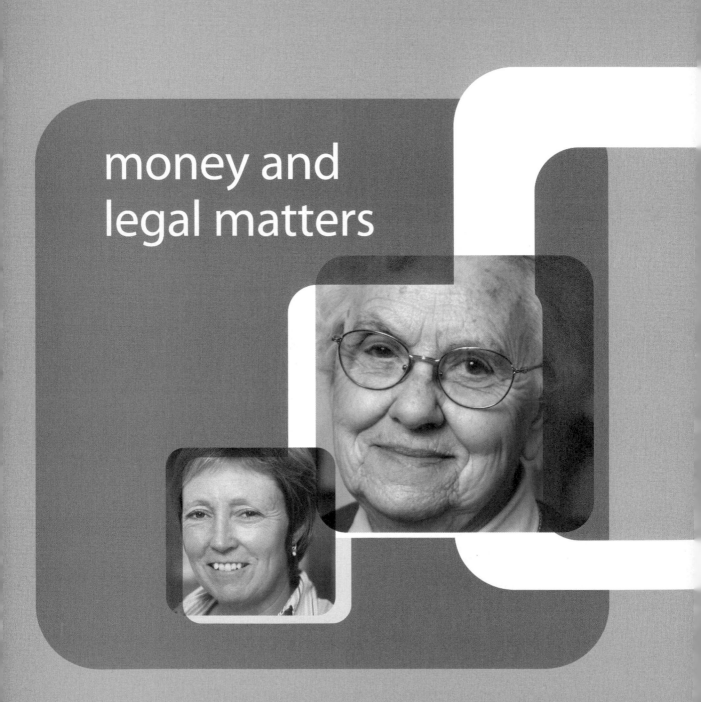

money and
legal matters

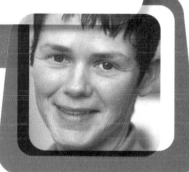

money and legal matters

Planning for the future

at a glance

- If the person is still able, encourage her to make arrangements for the future.
- Arrange to pay bills automatically.
- Encourage the person to grant powers of attorney if she can.
- Encourage the person to write a will if she can.

When you find out that someone you are close to has dementia, it can be very upsetting. Often practical arrangements for the future are the last thing you and the person may think about. But if the person with dementia is still able to, it is important to try to make plans sooner rather than later. People in the middle to later stages of dementia are likely not to be able to make legal arrangements any more. To make legal arrangements for the future, the person needs to be mentally capable of making her own decisions and legally able to sign documents. She should check with her doctor if she or her solicitor is not sure.

If the person is still able to do so, she should make some important decisions as soon as possible. She should:

- choose one or more people to look after her financial affairs and welfare decisions if she becomes unable to, and give them **power of attorney**

- make a **will**

- make sure you and the doctor know of any wishes about medical care in the future – she could write this down as an **advance directive** or **'living will'.**

More information is in the booklet *Dementia: Money and legal matters* – call the Dementia Helpline on **0808 808 3000** for a free copy.

What you can do

1. Encourage the person to see a solicitor to make powers of attorney covering her financial and welfare matters as soon as possible. That way she can decide who she trusts to make important decisions on her behalf in the future, if she becomes unable to manage. She will only be able to make a power of attorney if the solicitor is satisfied that she understands what she is doing and is not under pressure from anyone else. She can:

   - choose just one person or give two (or more) people joint power of attorney

   - choose the same or different people to handle her financial and welfare matters

   - choose substitutes in case her first choice can't carry on managing her affairs.

2. Encourage the person to make a will through her lawyer as soon as possible, so that she can choose what happens to her money and possessions. A will is only valid if made when the person is clearly aware of what she is doing, so it is important not to put it off.

3. Encourage the person to think about any wishes about medical care in the future and write these down as an advance directive or 'living will'. Make sure her doctor gets a copy.

4. If the person has no bank account, encourage her to open one.

5. Arrange direct debits so that the bank pays bills automatically. Gas, electricity and telephone companies and other organisations can help with this.

Managing everyday money matters for the person

at a glance

- Make sure the person has some cash.

- Start using the power of attorney if the person has made one.

- You can apply to access money in the person's bank account on her behalf.

- Keep the person's money separate from your own.

As time goes on, the person will become less able to cope with money. She may forget to pay bills, pay them twice, give money away or lose it. She is likely to lose her understanding of the value of money. For many people with dementia financial matters can be a great worry.

In time, you or someone else may have to take on more of the responsibility for managing her money.

What you can do

1. Make sure the person always has some cash, even if it is a small amount. This may reassure her and help her keep some independence.

2. Discuss the situation with the person with dementia as much as possible. Try to agree safeguards, such as making sure she doesn't have large amounts of money in the house.

3. If the person with dementia loses money, gives it away or forgets that she has

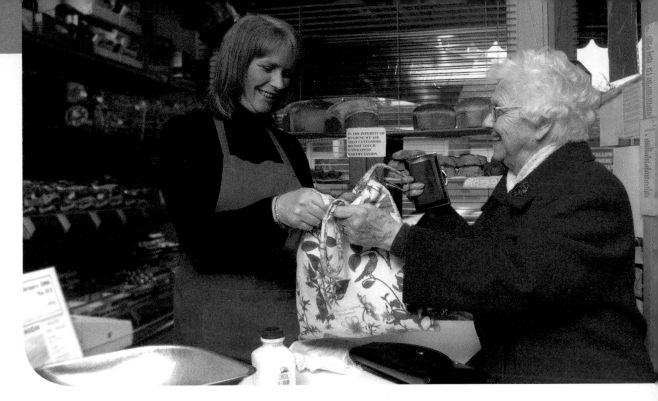

spent it, she may mistakenly accuse others of taking it. This can be distressing, but it is because of the illness. Reassure the person that she has enough money.

4. In some cases, unscrupulous people may take advantage of someone who is vulnerable because of dementia, so don't always assume that the person is mistaken if she feels money has been taken. You may need to investigate. If you feel that someone is stealing from her, involve the police and/or the social work department.

5. If you or someone else has a power of attorney for the person covering financial matters, make sure it is registered with the Public Guardian (see **Further information** on page 106). Once it is registered, you (or the person named as her attorney) can use it to manage the person's finances as if you were her.

6. If you are concerned that someone is misusing the person's money, for example using a power of attorney, the Public Guardian can investigate.

7. If the person has money in a joint bank or building society account, for example with her partner, in most cases the other account-holder can continue to use the account as usual.

8. If the person has money in an account in her sole name, and she is no longer able to manage it, you can apply to access the money yourself to spend it on her behalf. (But you can't do this if someone has a financial power of attorney for the person.) You don't need a solicitor to apply. You can get an application form for **Authority to Access Funds** from the Dementia Helpline or the Public Guardian. On the form you say what you need to spend each week or month on the person's bills, food, clothing and other items. You send it with a small fee to the Public Guardian.

9. If you handle the person's money, always keep it separate from your own. Keep a record of what you receive and spend, in case someone asks you to account for it.

More legal powers to help the person

at a glance

- Sometimes you may need more legal powers to make decisions for the person.

- The court can appoint a guardian or grant an intervention order.

In some cases, the court may have to give someone extra powers to manage the person's affairs. This may happen especially when no one has power of attorney for the person, and he or she is no longer able to make one. Perhaps the person needs someone to look after his or her finances or welfare long term. Or sometimes there may be a power of attorney but it doesn't give enough powers; for example, to sell the person's house.

Under the Adults with Incapacity Act, there are two ways the court can help. It can appoint a **guardian**, with financial or welfare powers or both, to look after the person's affairs. Or it can grant an **intervention order**, for a one-off decision or action.

What you can do

1. Call the Dementia Helpline or see the booklet *Dementia: Money and legal matters* (see **Further information** on pages 104 and 107) for more information.

2. See a solicitor, who can apply for guardianship or an intervention order for you. Alternatively, you can apply to the court yourself. If you decide to do it yourself, you can get more information and the forms you need from the Scottish Government Justice Department (see **Further information** on page 106).

3. The person with dementia may be entitled to Legal Aid.

Welfare benefits

at a glance

- You have a right to apply for benefits.

- Not all benefits are only available to people on low incomes.

- You can get advice and help filling in forms.

- Attendance allowance (for people over 65) and disability living allowance (for people under 65) help with care needs.

- Pension credit (for people over 60) and income support (for people under 60) help people on low incomes.

- Carers who care for more than 35 hours a week can apply for carer's allowance.

- People with dementia and carers liable to pay rent or council tax may be able to get help.

Caring for a person with dementia at home can be quite costly. Your income may have reduced because of your caring responsibilities. And there may be extra costs, such as more heating. Financial benefits may be available, both for the person with dementia and for you as the carer. Don't hesitate to claim – remember, you have a right to apply for benefits. It is a good idea to get advice to make sure you are applying for everything you and the person with dementia may be entitled to. Your local Citizens Advice Bureau or welfare benefits service can help.

Some benefits forms are very long. They may ask for a lot of detail about the help the person needs. Get help filling in the form if you can. Ask your local Alzheimer Scotland, Citizens Advice Bureau or carers' centre for help. Or use the Benefits Enquiry Line, who can fill forms in for you over the telephone (see **Further information**, page 102).

If the person does not get a benefit you have applied for, appeal. Appeals often succeed. Don't make a new claim, because it won't be backdated.

Benefits from the Department for Work and Pensions

1. Apply for these benefits from the Pension Service (if you are 60 or over), Jobcentre Plus (for those under 60) or Disability and Carers' Service (for attendance allowance, disability allowance and carer's allowance) – see under Department for Work and Pensions in **Further information** on page 104.

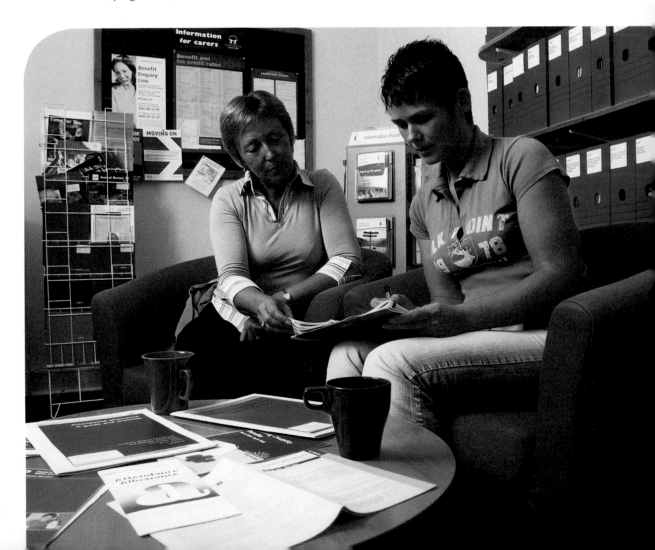

2. If the person with dementia needs care or supervision, she may qualify for attendance allowance (if she is over 65) or disability living allowance (if she is under 65). These two benefits do not depend on the person's income. They are paid at different rates according to the person's needs. Give as much detail on the form about the person's needs as you can. For example, if the person is not safe alone, give examples of what has happened or might happen.

3. If the person is under 65, apply as soon as possible for disability living allowance. This is because it can help with both care needs and mobility needs. Attendance allowance, for people over 65, does not help with mobility needs. If the person gets disability living allowance, she will still get it even when she passes 65. Someone who gets disability living allowance to help with mobility needs may be exempt from road tax if a car is registered in her name, even if someone else does the driving.

4. Carers who are over 16 and who look after someone who is eligible for attendance allowance or the middle or higher rate of disability living allowance (or some other benefits) for more than 35 hours a week can get carer's allowance. However, if you already get another benefit for the same amount or more you may not be able to receive it. But you might get extra money added to another benefit, such as income support, income-based jobseekers' allowance, pension credit, housing benefit or council tax benefit, instead. You can't get carer's allowance if you earn more than a certain limit. Check with your disability benefit centre (see **Further information**, Department for Work and Pensions, page 104).

5. Income support can be paid to some people who are under 60 and are not able to work, including people with health problems, a disability or who are caring for someone else. You can claim income support even if you are working as long as you are working less than 16 hours a week. If you have a partner you can claim as long as the one who claims works less than 16 hours and the other partner for not more than 24 hours a week. To get income support your income and savings must fall below certain levels.

6. Pension credit is for people aged 60 or over. It is more generous than income support and many more people qualify. Pension credit guarantees everyone aged 60 and over a minimum income, with more money for people over 65 who have saved for their retirement. Pension credit has two parts, the 'guarantee credit' and the 'savings credit'. Some people will get one or the other and some will get both.

7. You or the person with dementia may be entitled to other benefits, such as a community care grant from the social fund. Ask for a benefits check from your social work department benefits advisor or your local Citizens Advice Bureau.

8. You can collect the person's pension and other benefits if she authorises you. If she can't sign or doesn't understand what she is signing, ask the Department for Work and Pensions (DWP) to make you (or someone else) her appointee. As appointee, you can apply for and collect all benefits on behalf of the person. You must tell the DWP if the person's situation changes.

9. The DWP usually pays the pensions and benefits directly into a bank account. This can be useful, especially if the person's bills are paid by direct debit or standing order. If the person with dementia does not have a bank account he or she may be able to open a Post Office Card Account.

   The current contract for the Post Office Card Account runs out in 2010. It is not yet known if any other account will replace it.

   If the person is not able to operate an account, she may have granted someone power of attorney (see page 28) and this person can manage the account. Alternatively, you could apply to the Public Guardian to access the person's funds (see page 30). The DWP may suggest that the person's appointee has the benefits paid into his or her own account, but this may lead to problems, for example if the appointee is taken ill. A better solution is to ask the DWP for the Exception Service, so that the person is sent a cheque every week or fortnight.

Benefits from the council

1. People with dementia and carers liable to pay rent or council tax may be able to get help. Ask the local council for details.

2. If the person is 'severely mentally impaired', she may get a discount on the council tax, or an exemption. Most people with moderate to severe dementia will count as severely mentally impaired. Some carers can get a discount too. Getting a discount does not depend on your income. People on a low income may get council tax benefit, whether or not they also get a discount.

3. People on a low income may qualify for housing benefit for help with their rent.

4. People who receive the guarantee credit of pension credit are automatically entitled to full housing and council tax benefit, although they still need to complete the claim form.

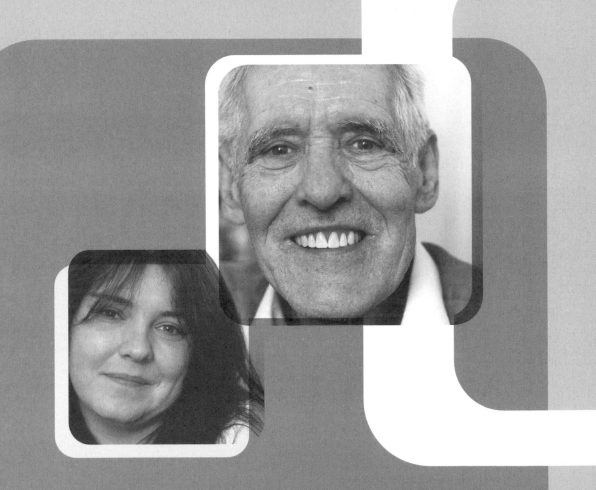

practical caring

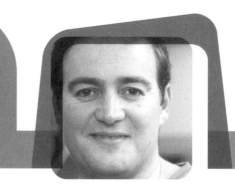

practical caring

Every person with dementia is different, and will be affected differently by the illness. This section looks at some of the challenges and problems you and the person with dementia may face.

Remember, not every problem will happen to any one person. Remember too that things will change as the illness progresses. A difficulty which seems impossible to solve may just disappear with time.

There is a great deal that you can do to make things better for yourself and the person with dementia. The **What you can do** sections list some practical ways of dealing with the changes which people with dementia go through. Finding the best way of coping is often a matter of trial and error. But these ideas have helped other carers.

As much as possible, support the person with dementia to keep doing things for herself, rather than taking over. This can take patience, but it will help the person to maintain her skills and independence. It can be tempting just to do something yourself because it is quicker and easier, but it is important to let the person keep doing what she can still do. Use prompts and reminders to help her. But don't feel bad if this isn't always possible. Sometimes you will have to balance the extra time and patience needed to help the person do something with the benefit of doing it yourself more quickly.

Don't feel you have to cope on your own. Talk to the person's doctor, community psychiatric nurse or occupational therapist and to other carers. Or call the 24-hour Dementia Helpline for suggestions on how to approach a problem.

> *For a while my mother kept losing her purse. She would get very upset and accuse me or her home help of stealing it. But she has become much calmer over the last few months. She doesn't look for her purse at all any more.*

Looking after the person

Each person with dementia is an individual and has her own lifestyle and experiences. Try to remember this when you are caring. Try to help the person to carry on with existing interests and social activities as much as possible.

Physical well-being

at a glance

- Keeping well physically is just as important for someone with dementia as for anyone else.

- Physical illnesses can make dementia symptoms worse.

- Try to make sure the person has a healthy diet and enough physical activity.

- Make sure she sees the doctor if she becomes unwell.

It is important to make sure the person with dementia stays as healthy as possible. A healthy diet and enough exercise are important for maintaining physical health and can help to avoid illness.

Problems with seeing or hearing can make life extra difficult for someone with dementia. Illnesses such as infections can make the symptoms of dementia worse, and the person may be more confused until the illness is treated. Avoiding constipation is important too, because it can cause discomfort and pain.

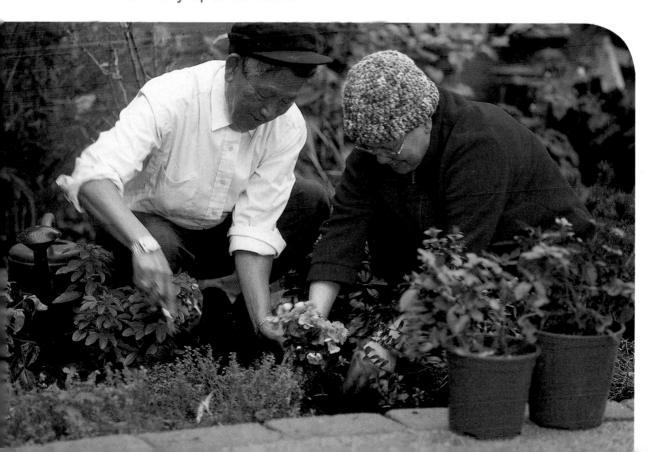

It may be difficult for the person with dementia to tell you if there is something wrong. If the person seems irritable, or more confused, it may be because she is uncomfortable or in pain.

What you can do

1. Try to make sure the person eats a healthy diet, with plenty of fruit and vegetables, and foods such as whole grain bread which are high in fibre, to help avoid constipation. Ask for advice from her doctor or nurse.

2. Make sure she drinks enough. She may not realise she is thirsty, so you may need to keep reminding her, or prompting her by offering her the cup or glass. It is important she does not get dehydrated, as this could make her constipated, exhausted and more confused. Aim for about 6–8 cups or glasses a day. A few cups of tea and coffee are fine, but try to make sure she also drinks plenty of water, juice or milk as well.

3. Exercise is important, and may also help her to sleep better. Try to make sure she does something active every day, even if it's just a walk to the shops.

> *When I started visiting my uncle I was shocked because he hardly understood a word I said. It was several weeks before I realised that he often forgot to put his hearing aid in, or turn it on. With it working, he was much better – still very forgetful, but at least now I could remind him about things.*

4. If she has problems with her eyesight or hearing, talk to her doctor, optician or hearing specialist. It is important that she can see or hear as well as possible so that she can take in what's going on around her – poor hearing or vision can make it much harder for someone with dementia to cope.

5. Make sure she sees her doctor if she is ill (for example with a chest or bladder infection), has a fall, becomes constipated or if she seems in pain or depressed. All these can affect people with dementia just as much as anyone else, and can be treated. Without treatment, they may make the symptoms of dementia worse. She should also see the doctor if she develops hallucinations (seeing things which are not there).

Mental stimulation

at a glance

- **People with dementia need interesting and enjoyable things to do.**
- **The right activities can help the person to maintain her abilities and independence.**
- **Try to help the person keep doing things she used to do.**
- **Activities need to be suitable for the individual.**
- **Friends and family can enjoy helping with activities.**

Like anyone else, someone with dementia needs things to do, for interest, enjoyment and satisfaction and to have a good quality of life. Without enough to do, people can get bored and frustrated. Staying as mentally active as possible

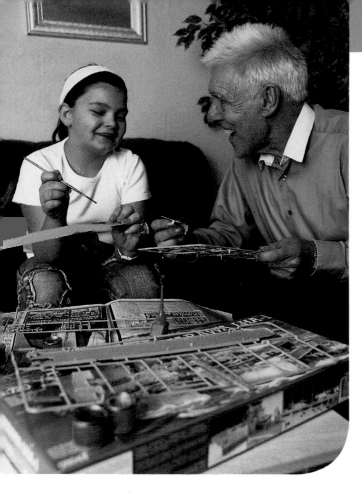

different activities at different times, according to how she is feeling. You may have to help more with an activity, or simplify it, as time goes on.

Try to find activities which won't risk her feeling she has failed at something. A feeling of failure can be very distressing.

Don't feel you must provide something to do every minute of the day. Quiet time is important too. Sometimes the job of caring for someone with dementia takes up so much time and energy that it's hard to fit in enjoyable activities. Try to find help with caring so that you are under less pressure. A day centre can offer enjoyable and stimulating activities for the person and give you time for yourself. See **Getting help**, on page 79.

Call the Dementia Helpline on **0808 808 3000** for a free copy of Alzheimer Scotland's booklet *Activities: A guide for carers of people with dementia*, which will help give you some ideas.

> *My mother loves to dust. She sometimes does the mantelpiece over and over again, but she gets a lot of satisfaction out of it, so I don't stop her.*

What you can do

1. Think about what the person used to enjoy for ideas on what to try. Help her to keep doing things she used to do.

2. Involve family and friends – for example, perhaps they would like to accompany the person on outings, help her to stay involved in family life and with community events, play a game or read the paper with her.

can help the person to maintain her abilities and be as independent as she can. Stimulating activities can help to keep her mentally alert, so she may manage better, although doing activities can't affect the underlying illness.

Because of the illness, thinking of what to do, getting started and maintaining concentration all get harder. People may become withdrawn and lose their confidence. They are likely to need a lot more encouragement. You can help by helping the person you care for find activities she will enjoy and things you can enjoy together.

Each person with dementia will enjoy different activities, according to her interests and how the illness affects her. The person you care for will enjoy

3. Break down tasks into more manageable steps so that the person can do the parts she is still able to cope with. For example, if she can no longer make a cup of tea, suggest that she gets the cups out while you put the kettle on, and so on.

4. Many people with dementia can still remember things that happened a long time ago, even if they can't remember more recent events. So they may enjoy activities like looking through old family photographs or copies of old newspapers, for example.

> *My father used to go down to the bowling club every week. He stopped going for a while because he was worried that his pals wouldn't accept him because he has Alzheimer's disease. When he told me I asked if he minded me talking to them. He said that was OK, and a couple of them still come round every week and drive him there.*

5. The person may enjoy gardening, knitting, sewing or DIY. Try not to take over, but to help with each stage of an activity as she needs it.

6. Activities needn't be complicated. Many people with dementia like to feel useful, and may enjoy helping around the house.

7. Many people will enjoy listening to familiar music.

8. Remember that even if the person doesn't remember an activity, it is still worthwhile if she enjoys it at the time.

> *Until she had her first stroke, my sister used to be an avid bridge player. She still loves to play cards, so now we play snap and other simple games.*

Life story book

at a glance

- Making a life story book can be enjoyable, both for the person and for you.
- Looking at the book will help the person reminisce later.
- It can help other people involved in her care get to know about her and what is important to her.
- The book is also a record for you of the person's life.

A life story book is a collection of reminders of important times in the person's life, such as photographs, tickets, postcards and so on. A life story book can be enjoyable to make and can benefit the person in many ways. Most people can still remember a lot about their past even when their recent memory is very poor. Making a life story book is an opportunity for the person to talk about herself and her life.

The person may enjoy just looking through the book later. And the book can help family, friends and staff to get to know the person, her life and what is important to her.

A life story book can be important for carers and families too. It is your chance to find out things about the person's life you may never have known about before, and to record the person's past. When the person can no longer tell you her stories, you will have something to help you remember.

What you can do

1. Use a scrapbook or photograph album to make the life story book.

2. Help the person look through old photographs, postcards, tickets and other reminders of her past. Help her choose which ones she would like to put into her book.

3. Talk with her about the things she chooses, so that you can label the items together.

4. Put in notes and anecdotes, for example about her parents, childhood, school, work, relationships, children, friends, homes, hobbies and holidays.

5. Ask her about things she feels strongly about, from food and drink to music, sports or politics, and put in reminders of these.

6. Ask for her permission to show the book to other people, such as family members, friends and staff who are involved in her care.

> *My sister had six children and she'd kept locks of their baby hair, so we put them in. We also included a scrap of material from cushion covers she'd made years ago out of the curtains of her first house, and every time she looks at that page she tells a story about those curtains and how she loved them so much she couldn't throw the material out when they were done.*

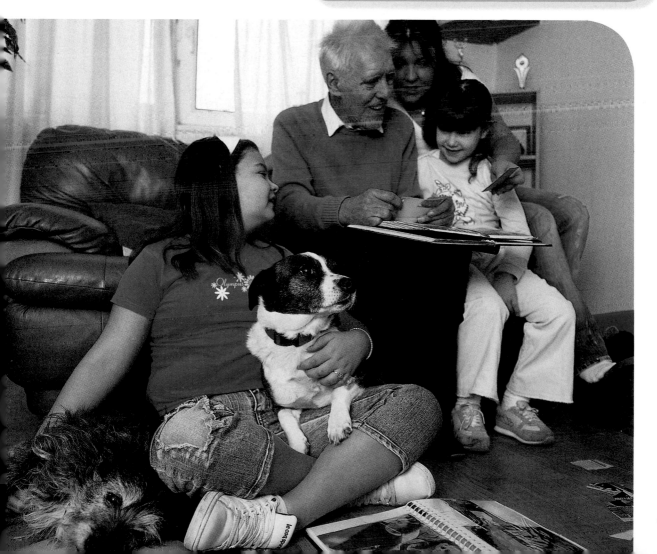

Spiritual well-being

at a glance

- Find out what used to be important to the person.
- Try to help her to keep attending religious worship.
- Help the person to stay in contact with other people and newsletters from her place of worship.
- Help the person with personal devotion.
- Ask for pastoral care.

Caring for the whole person with dementia means caring for spiritual needs too. Most people's spirituality is to do with their ethnic culture, tradition and upbringing. A person's individual awareness of her place and purpose in creation is unique. This is the person's spirituality. People have different personal ways of finding a sense of spiritual well-being. If spirituality has been important to someone, it is important to help her to have contact with things that in the past were part of her spiritual well-being. Without this, some people may feel abandoned. They may feel a sense of loss of worth and purpose.

Although my aunt doesn't speak any more, she still loves to sing hymns and remembers every word.

What you can do

1. Find out what spiritual things if any used to be important to the person. For example, this may include religious worship, meditation, books, songs or chants, symbols, places or other things.

2. If the person attended religious worship or groups or festivals, try to help her to keep attending for as long as possible. If this becomes impossible, perhaps she can continue to take part in worship at home.

3. Help the person to stay in contact with other people from her place of worship. Encourage visitors.

4. Help the person to feel that she still belongs, for example by reading newsletters or magazines from the church, mosque, synagogue, temple or other place of worship.

5. Help the person with personal devotion. For example, familiar readings from holy books, prayers or meditation.

6. Ask the person's minister, priest, rabbi, imam or other religious leader or teacher to visit to give pastoral care to the person, and to you if you wish.

Loss of mental abilities

Forgetfulness

at a glance

- Keep to routines and don't make changes unless you have to.

- Use memory aids and draw attention to them.

- Drop reminders into your conversation.

- Use familiar objects and photographs as reminders.

Most people with dementia will have memory problems, which become more severe as the illness progresses. For mild memory problems, simple memory aids may be very helpful. Later in the illness memory aids probably won't help. You will need to give more direct reminders and help. The person with dementia may become more confused and 'lost' or disorientated. She may forget basic facts such as who other people are, where they are and what year it is. She may confuse the past with the present.

Early on in the illness there are simple practical ways to jog the person's memory. The following ideas will help you and the person with dementia cope with forgetfulness.

> *Sometimes my Dad would mention a visitor he'd had, but he was never sure who it was. So I put out a 'visitor's book' and asked people to sign in. It turned out that the mystery person was his care worker.*

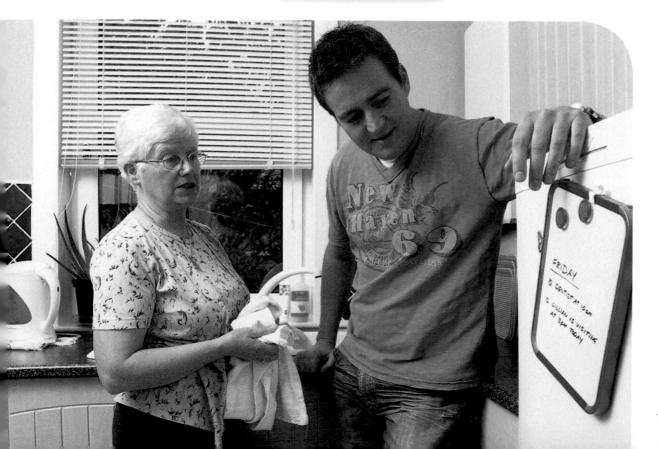

They will help the person keep her mind alert for as long as possible. This approach is known as reality orientation. It means providing reminders to help the person keep an idea of where she is, who people are, what time of day it is, what season it is and so on.

Reassurance is very important. The person may be aware that she now can't remember what she used to. This can be upsetting, frightening and frustrating. Try to be reassuring. Respond to the emotions the person shows as well as to what she actually says or does.

> *To help my brother keep track of time, I'll usually drop something into the conversation like, 'Oh good – it's Saturday – but isn't it cold for October!'.*

What you can do

1. Keep to routines as much as you can and try not to change where things are. Being in familiar surroundings helps. Changes can make confusion worse.

2. Memory aids work best when the person is in the habit of using them; for example, if she has always used a diary. Try to help her get into the habit as early as you can in the illness. Get other people who visit to write in the diary too. You can use it as a reminder for her of what she has been doing.

3. Get a large clock with the day and date. A loud tick helps remind the person with dementia where the clock is. Put up a calendar and mark off the days.

> *Whenever I go out I leave a note for my wife on the door of the fridge to say when I'll be back. Before I go I point it out to her and get her to read it to me by asking if she can read my writing, just to make sure she understands.*

4. Put signs in words or pictures on doors to help the person find the way around. Or just leave doors open so that the person can see what's in each room.

5. Use a memory board or notice board as a reminder of what is going on. Put it somewhere it is easy to see, such as in the kitchen.

6. You will need to draw the person's attention to memory aids and check that she understands them. The aids alone don't work. Remind her to look at the memory board, calendar, diary and signs. Leave notes where the person will see them if she is still able to understand them.

7. If you are not with the person, try reminding her about things by phoning.

8. You may need to provide basic facts in your conversation such as reminders about time, place and people. Helpful facts might include who you are, where she is, where you are going, what is happening and so on. Be tactful and don't wait for the person to fail.

9. Family photographs, including photographs of the person with dementia, can help her keep a sense of identity. Talk about them, particularly if her sight is not good. Named photos of regular visitors (family, friends, home help) may help her to know people when they call.

> *My sister gets anxious sometimes and wants to go home to look after her children. She's forgotten that they're grown up with children of their own now.*

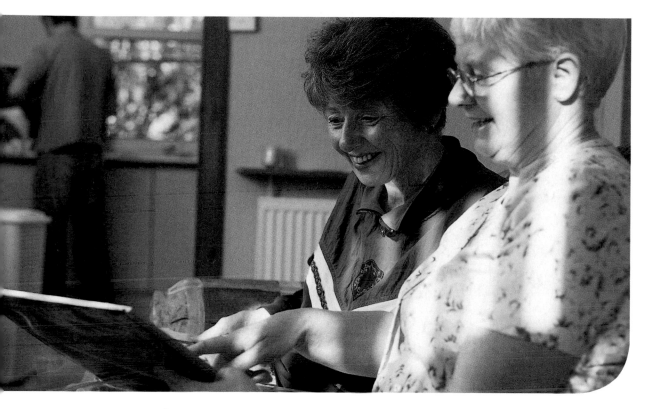

Repeated questions

at a glance

- Remember that repeated questions are not meant to annoy you: they need repeated answers.

- Try to be patient, tactful and reassuring.

- Try other ways of reminding the person of the answer, such as a notebook.

- Try to change the subject gently.

- Keep the person with dementia involved in what is happening.

Some people with dementia keep asking the same question over and over again. This is because the person does not remember asking or can't remember the answer. Many carers find this very difficult to deal with. It can be frustrating and irritating, especially if the person follows you around the house asking questions. The person may seem afraid to let you out of her sight. This is because she may not be able to remember where you are or whether you will be back.

> *He used to ask the same thing again and again and it used to drive me round the bend sometimes. It was usually about when the bus for the day centre was coming, what time was dinner, things like that. So now I try to remind him about things as I talk, and I put up reminders on the fridge door. He still asks, but not as often. I can either answer or just point to the fridge. It helps me keep my patience longer.*

What you can do

1. Remind yourself that the person really does forget having asked a question before, or forgets the answer. Remember that she is not doing it deliberately to annoy you.

2. Be tactful. For example it is better to say, 'Oh, didn't I mention that we're going to the shops to buy bread and milk', rather than 'I've told you that already'.

> *The best way I found to keep calm was to see how many different ways I could answer the same question.*

3. Be reassuring, The person may be asking because she is anxious about something. Try reassuring her physically, perhaps with a hug.

4. If the person can still understand written reminders, try writing the answer to the question in a notebook or on a notice board. Point it out as you answer. Try to help the person get used to looking there for the answer.

5. Keep the person involved in what is happening. Make eye contact when you talk to her. Remember to include the person with dementia if there is a group conversation. This will help lessen anxiety and may reduce questions.

6. Use memory aids (see page 45).

7. Try to divert her attention and involve her in another activity.

8. Even with all your efforts she may keep repeating questions. Sometimes you may have to leave the room to keep your patience.

Conversation and communication

at a glance

- Check dentures, hearing aids and glasses.
- Face the person, speak clearly and use simple sentences.
- Be patient and allow extra time.
- Help with word-finding problems.
- Use touch and gesture.
- Let the person know that you understand how frustrating it is.
- You may have to repeat yourself slightly differently.
- Use simple questions.
- Try not to embarrass the person.

As dementia gets worse communication becomes a problem. You may find that the person seems deaf at times. Deafness may be the problem, but it is also likely that the person hears but does not understand. Dementia slows people down in their ability to take things in and make sense of what they hear. Some people may have difficulty finding the right words for what they want to say. They may also begin to lose track of what they are saying in the middle of a sentence. It becomes harder to hold a conversation. This can be very frustrating for both people with dementia and carers.

What you can do

1. Make sure that the person's dentures, glasses or hearing aid are in good working order and are the correct prescription. Poor sight and hearing can make people more confused and conversation difficult.

2. Speak clearly, simply and slowly but don't shout. Make sure the person can see your face when you speak.

3. Try to get one idea across at a time.

4. You may have to repeat yourself. Sometimes it helps if you say things slightly differently the second time: 'Your sister Freda is coming to tea today.' 'We're having a visitor this afternoon. Your sister Freda is coming.'

5. Use questions which ask for a simple answer. Instead of asking my grandmother, 'What would you like to do this afternoon?', I'll say, 'Do you want to go for a walk, or shall we look at some photographs?'.

6. Allow plenty of time for the person to take in what you say and to reply.

7. Try not to confuse or embarrass the person by correcting her bluntly.

8. If the person with dementia cannot find the right words, ask her to describe what she means and suggest a word. But don't get into the habit of providing the right word as soon as she hesitates. If you do, she may become less confident. She might give up trying. Be encouraging but let her know you understand how frustrating it is trying to find the right words.

9. Guess what the person is trying to say. Always ask if your guess is right. This is especially important when you are trying to understand what the person feels. She may not be able to say why she feels worried, sad, angry or unhappy. If you do manage to grasp the feeling,

let her know this. It will help to lessen feelings of being alone and isolated.

10. A smile, touch or gesture can be just as important in getting the message across and showing that you care. Holding the person's hand when you talk can also be very reassuring.

11. Many people with dementia enjoy talking about the past. You may both enjoy reliving some of these memories together. Talking about things which she remembers well may help the person to feel secure. Try to make sure that she doesn't confuse these memories with the present. You can do this by making comparisons with how things were then and now. A life story book can be a useful aid (see page 42).

> *It was hard to know what was upsetting my husband. He wasn't able to say. Then at bed-time I noticed his toe was badly swollen.*

Confused thinking

at a glance

- Try not to go along with confused thinking, but be flexible.

- Sometimes gentle correction works.

- Use distraction.

- Talk about feelings the person is showing.

As dementia progresses the person's thinking becomes more mixed up. She may confuse memories of the past with the present. She may confuse facts with imaginings. As well as using memory aids, there are some good ways of trying to deal with confused thinking.

> *My partner sometimes gets mixed up about what year it is. Sometimes he goes back in his mind to when he was working and gets anxious about getting to work on time. The first few times I told him that he doesn't work any more but he'd insist he does and we'd end up arguing. So now I reassure him that it's all right, he doesn't have to go to work today.*

Dementia can cause difficulties with abstract thought as well as memory problems. For example, the person may find it harder to understand emotions or humour. She may take things literally.

> *I used to spend so long prompting my mother to dress herself that it became the main activity of the morning. Now we compromise. I help her a bit more, and with the time saved we go out for a walk or do something else we both enjoy.*

Don't agree with confused thinking. This can just make it worse. But you don't always have to try to put the person right. Use a flexible approach, depending on the situation.

What you can try

1. Try disagreeing tactfully to correct the confusion. No one likes to be corrected too often, so you have to be careful with this approach. Sometimes it can be upsetting for the person. You will have to play it by ear.

2. Don't confront the person. Try diverting her onto another subject until she forgets.

3. Respond kindly to the person's feelings without agreeing with what she is saying.

> *'Another beautiful day,' my mother would say on coming down for breakfast – often with the rain lashing down! And I would simply say, 'You're feeling good then?'*

Daily living

People with dementia usually find everyday tasks such as dressing or eating gradually harder as time goes on. So they need more help. If you can, try to help the person with dementia to do things rather than doing them yourself. This can take more time, but it helps the person keep as independent as possible. You may have to find a balance between time and effort for you and independence for the person.

Dressing

at a glance

- Allow plenty of time.
- Don't do too much for the person – encourage independence.
- Lay out clothes in the order the person is used to.
- Allow choice – but you may need to limit it.
- Gently correct any errors in dressing.
- Explain what you are doing when you give help.
- If necessary, alter clothing to make dressing easier.

People with dementia often have problems with dressing. They may lose track of the order of putting on clothes or forget half-way through and start to undress. They may struggle with fastenings and give up easily. The person may need help but not want it. For all these reasons dressing can take a long time.

What you can do

1. Allow plenty of time for the person to get dressed. If rushed she may become more confused and upset. Make sure the room is warm and she has used the toilet first.

2. As a general rule avoid doing too much for the person. Encourage her to do things for herself. This will help keep up self-esteem and confidence. Remind her what to do next if necessary. If that doesn't work, try showing her with actions. Break things down into small steps.

3. Allow the person some choice, even if it is limited.

4. Lay out clothes in the order she will put them on. If possible, keep to the order that the person was in the habit of using.

> *When my Dad saw all his shirts in the cupboard he just couldn't choose and got confused and upset. So I put most of them in a different place and just left him a couple of his favourites. Now he picks the shirt he's going to wear quite happily.*

5. If the person tries to put something on the wrong way, tactfully correct her and give help. Explain what you are doing. The more patient you can be the less likely the person is to become irritable and uncooperative.

6. If you have to do most of the dressing for the person, start by putting clothes on either the top or bottom half of her body, then the other half. Don't at any time leave her entirely naked.

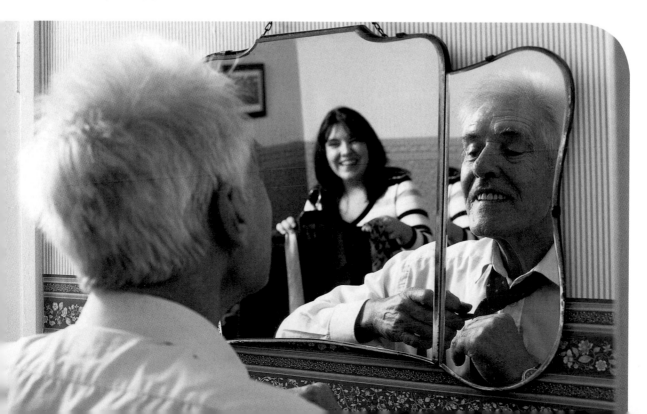

7. If the person has had a stroke, this may have left a weakness in a limb. It is much easier to place the weak limb into an item of clothing first and take it out last.

8. Buttons and hooks may be difficult. You can often replace them with zips or Velcro. Bras are easier to manage if they fasten at the front. Consider self-support stockings or socks.

9. If the person is incontinent and needs a great deal of help with dressing, some carers find that track suit tops and trousers can be very useful. They are practical, easy to change, quick to wash and dry and they don't need ironing. But they are not right for everyone – some people with dementia may not feel comfortable or dignified in clothes that are different to what they normally wore. For information about special designs of clothing, contact the Dementia Helpline on **0808 808 3000.**

10. The person should only wear slippers for short times. Well-fitting shoes give support and reduce the risk of foot problems.

11. Put clothes for washing out of sight so that the person does not put them on again.

> *Every time I visited my mother she was wearing exactly the same clothes. She had plenty of other things in her wardrobe but she wouldn't wear them. We'd argue when I tried to get her to change. So I bought some more clothes the same as the ones she likes. She doesn't notice when I put out the clean ones while she's in bed. Now she's cleaner and we're both more relaxed because I've stopped nagging her.*

Appearance and personal care

at a glance

- Compliment the person when she looks good.
- Remind the person about cleaning teeth or shaving.
- Show the person what to do if she gets mixed up.
- Encourage men to get used to an electric shaver early in the illness.
- Keep up regular dental and hair appointments.

In time dementia causes the person to forget how to do even basic tasks of personal care. She may forget to clean her teeth or brush her hair. Cutting nails may be a problem and men may have difficulty with shaving. Some people with dementia lose interest in how they look. Of course, many people with dementia do not like to be reminded about these personal tasks. But it is important to encourage the person to do as much as possible for herself.

> *My brother will rarely open his mouth to let me brush his back teeth. But he usually lets me brush the front ones.*

My mother gets a great boost from her fortnightly trip to the hairdresser. I also try to make sure she has a touch of make-up and nail varnish. She always used to wear it and I think it makes her feel more self-confident.

What you can do

1. Take notice and compliment the person when she looks good. When she needs help or prompting, be tactful. Criticism or nagging is likely to upset her.

2. Remind the person when necessary about cleaning teeth. It may help if you clean your teeth at the same time to remind her what to do. You may need to clean the person's teeth or dentures as her illness gets worse.

3. Dental care is vital. Ensure regular check-ups. Ask about the home dental service if visits to the dentist become too difficult. (Contact the health board if the person's own dentist is unable to visit.)

4. Remember to check finger and toe nails regularly. Cut them if the person can't. If you can't cut them arrange for a podiatrist (chiropodist) to visit (see page 89).

5. A trip to the hairdressers or a shampoo and set at home may help the person feel good. So can make-up and nail varnish.

6. Men may need to be reminded to shave each morning. Using an electric shaver is safer and may allow the person to shave himself independently for longer. Later in the illness he may find it hard to learn to use a new kind of razor. If he keeps using a traditional razor, you will need to supervise shaving. You may even have to do it for him.

Bathing

at a glance

- Supervise bathing as required.
- Make bath-time as pleasant as you can and give reassurance.
- Use bath aids to make bathing easier and safer.
- Ask for advice and help.

It may be difficult to persuade the person with dementia to have a bath. She may believe that she has recently taken one, when you know she hasn't. Bathing itself can have its problems. Some people forget how to wash themselves, wash one area several times and forget others, forget to use soap or forget to rinse off the soap. The person may not like being supervised.

My Dad hated me helping him in the bathroom, but there really wasn't an alternative. I told him that he did it for me when I was wee, and now it was my turn. I think he's got used to it now, and thinking of it that way made it easier for me.

Help with such intimate care can be difficult for both you and the person with dementia, especially if you are caring for someone such as a parent. Try talking about it with the person. Reassure her that you are there to help.

What you can do

1. Try to make bath-time as pleasant as possible. Allow plenty of time and ensure that the bathroom is warm. All sorts of little things might help to make bathing more relaxed. Try music or bubble bath, for example. If the person is unwilling to bath, it may help just to run a bath and offer it to her, rather than ask her about it beforehand.

2. Use a non-slip rubber mat in the bath and ensure that the flooring beside the bath is non-slip.

3. You may have to help the person in and out of the bath. Various aids may be available. A bath seat might help. Hand rails on the side of the bath make it easier for the person to get in and out. Ask the occupational therapist or nurse (see page 89).

4. Put a chair beside the bath for yourself.

5. If the person uses the bathroom alone, make sure the door can't be locked, or that the lock can be opened from outside in an emergency.

6. There are many new shower unit designs which some carers find useful. Ask the occupational therapist. But a shower may upset the person with dementia if she is not used to them.

7. Washing intimate areas of the body is important, but can feel embarrassing. Often this can feel especially awkward if you are helping a parent of the opposite sex. Try giving the person the cloth or sponge and guiding her hand. Some people find it easier to be bathed by someone they don't know, such as a nurse or care assistant.

8. If bathing is difficult or distressing, think about whether the person has to have a bath. Is it necessary for hygiene, or would an all-over wash do instead?

9. If you cannot deal with bathing or showering, for example if you and the person don't feel comfortable about it, or if you need to lift the person, ask your health visitor, doctor or social worker for advice. Sometimes the district nurse or a home care assistant may be able to call in and help. Different areas have different arrangements for bathing services. People who go to a day hospital may be able to have a bath there if bathing at home is not possible, and some day centres offer baths.

> *My Dad was very unwilling to have a bath. I think he was embarrassed for his daughter to see him naked. I talked to the day centre he goes to and they agreed to try. The staff had no problem at all persuading him to bath with their help.*

Managing continence

at a glance

- See the doctor first of all.
- Don't make a big issue of incontinence.
- Try occasional reminders or regular toileting.
- Agitation may mean that the person needs to go to the toilet.
- If buttons or zips cause problems, replace them with Velcro.
- Ask your community nurse about aids.
- Make sure the person knows how to get to the toilet.

- Avoid constipation with a good diet.
- Get help with laundry if available.
- Restrict drinks in the evening.
- Don't use an electric blanket for someone who is incontinent.
- Don't use laxatives unless the doctor has prescribed them.

Some people with dementia may become incontinent of urine (wet themselves). Bowel incontinence is not common until very late in the illness.

If the person becomes incontinent, don't just accept it as part of the illness. Often the person may not be truly incontinent at all. She may have forgotten the way to the toilet or how to recognise the toilet. Or she may not recognise the feeling of a full bladder. Helping the person may solve the problem.

Incontinence of urine may be the result of an infection or some physical problem. For instance, in men it may be caused by an enlarged prostate gland. Infections can be treated. Physical problems can often be put right. Consult the person's doctor or community nurse.

Sadly, sometimes incontinence is because of the degree of brain failure in dementia. In this case, it cannot be cured and slowly gets worse. In the end the person may need changes of clothes through the day and bed-linen at night. Ask the doctor if there is a continence adviser in your area and ask about incontinence aids. Call the Dementia Helpline for an information

sheet on continence management – see **Further information**, page 104.

What you can do

1. Consult the doctor about the problem. Ask for an explanation of the cause, after she has examined the person and done tests.

2. If the incontinence cannot be treated, ask for an assessment by the community nurse or continence adviser. The nurse or adviser can supply appropriate aids such as pads, pants and protective bedding. Don't just go out and buy your own supplies. The person is entitled to incontinence equipment if she has a medical need.

3. Make sure the nurse or adviser shows you how to use the products. If you don't use them properly they might not be very effective, which can be distressing.

4. Watch for any restlessness or agitation. These may be signs that the person needs to go to the toilet, but she may not realise this.

5. To reduce embarrassment, take a very matter-of-fact approach. Avoid making an issue out of the problem.

6. It may help if you remind the person to go to the toilet at regular intervals. The timing will vary from person to person. Try keeping a chart of when she needs the toilet to help work out a routine.

7. It may help to have a sign on the toilet door, or just to leave the door open so that she can see the toilet. Leave a light on at night to help the person find the way.

8. Zips or buttons may be too awkward for the person to manage. If this is a problem, clothes with Velcro fastenings might help.

9. If the toilet is not easy to get to, it may help to have a commode. Ask the community nurse.

10. It is dangerous for anyone who is incontinent to use a standard electric blanket.

11. Sometimes soiling is caused by severe constipation. Constipation may be caused by a poor diet. A well-balanced diet with plenty of fibre (roughage), such as fruit, vegetables, wholewheat bread and cereals helps prevent constipation. Make sure the person has enough to drink. This also helps prevent constipation. Don't use laxatives unless the doctor has prescribed them.

> *My mother would try every door looking for the toilet, so I put a notice on the door which said 'Ladies' and she had no problem finding it. But a friend who tried this said a picture of a lavatory worked best for his mother.*

12. In some areas there is a laundry service to help with soiled linen. Contact your local social work office.

Eating and drinking

at a glance

- Allow plenty of time for eating.
- Make sure dentures fit well.
- Say what meal it is and what they will be eating.
- Buy or make eating aids.
- Be patient with untidiness.
- See that the person gets a balanced diet and enough fluid.
- Use snacks and finger foods.
- Find out about meals on wheels.
- Ask the doctor or nurse for advice.

People with dementia may have poor appetite. They may not be very interested in eating. Some people with dementia seem to lose weight even when they are eating properly. They may be confused about whether they have eaten or not. Some want to start on the next meal as soon as they finish one. They may lose their table manners and become messy in their eating habits. They may have difficulty using cutlery. Eating certain foods can be a problem particularly if someone's dentures don't fit well.

> *My partner is so restless now that he can't seem to sit and finish a meal. But he's happy to take a sandwich and eat it as he goes.*

Too little to drink causes dehydration. This can cause constipation and make the person exhausted and more confused.

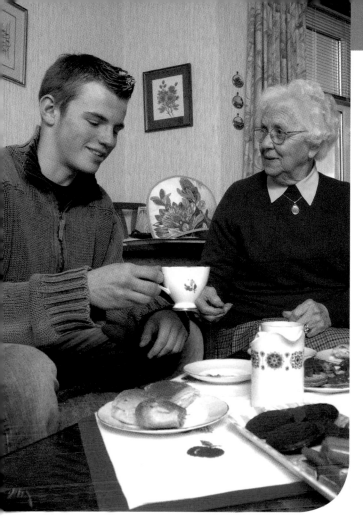

5. If weight loss is a problem put out snacks. If the person is restless, provide tasty finger foods so that she can eat and walk around at the same time.

6. See that the person gets enough to drink. She needs at least 8 cups of fluid a day. This can include soup and fruit juice as well as tea and coffee. Make sure that drinks are not too hot. Avoid too much fluid just before going to bed.

7. If the person has dentures, check that they are in place and fit properly.

8. Make forks and spoons easier to grasp by wrapping the handles to make them thicker. If forks are difficult, the person may be happier using a spoon. You may also need to use a spill-proof cup. You can use an ordinary cup with cling film over the top and a straw inserted in it. Ask your health visitor or occupational therapist about other eating aids.

9. Try having the main meal in the middle of the day. This may help reduce night-time indigestion and discomfort. It may also help the person sleep better.

10. If the person will only eat certain foods, check with the doctor that her diet is healthy.

11. For people living alone, or alone during the day, ask the social work department about meals on wheels. Try leaving out cold food such as ham, cheese, sandwiches or flasks of hot food. Don't leave cans and packets which are hard to open. However, the person may not eat food that you leave for her. If this is a problem, perhaps a home help could come in at lunch time to make sure the person eats. Ask the social work department.

12. If someone loses weight despite eating well, or seems to have lost her appetite, consult the doctor. It may be due to dementia or to another medical problem.

What you can do

1. Allow plenty of time for meals. Make sure meal times are pleasant and enjoyable.

2. Tell the person which meal it is and what there is to eat. You may have to remind the person how to eat by prompting her to pick up the fork or spoon.

3. As far as possible avoid feeding someone who has difficulty. This encourages the person to be more dependent than necessary. But sometimes spoon feeding may be needed.

4. Try not to worry too much about table manners. Allow the person to feed herself even if it is messy. Plastic table cloths are very practical.

Psychological problems

Apathy and loss of interest

at a glance

- Plan something of interest each day.
- Involve the person with dementia in planning as far as you can.
- Encourage the person to do tasks around the house.
- Get friends to help.
- Accept that some loss of interest is bound to happen. You don't have to fight it all the time!

People with dementia often seem to become bored and withdrawn. They may not seem able to keep an interest in anything for more than a few minutes. This can be upsetting if you are used to seeing the person you care for busy and happy.

Over the last year, my mother has found it very hard to get herself organised to do things. She tends just to sit in her chair most of the day if left to herself. But I've found that she'll enjoy doing things like sorting out the sewing box as long as I get her started.

Some people with dementia may be depressed. This can be treated. If you think the person you care for is depressed, seek medical advice. But even without depression, apathy is common in dementia.

What you can do

1. Try to make sure that each day has something of interest for the person with dementia. It might be going for a walk, listening to favourite music, a game of cards, gardening; anything which the person enjoys. See **Mental stimulation** on page 40 for ideas.

2. Involve the person with dementia as far as possible in choosing what to do.

3. Talk about the day's activities.

4. Help the person with dementia do whatever jobs around the house she can manage. Doing these tasks can help the person to feel useful – even if you have to go over the work again later yourself!

5. Try to get other people involved. A chat with old friends, perhaps talking about the past, can help to raise the person's spirits. Old friends will soon get used to the changes in the person and make allowances.

6. Remember that a time to be quiet, sit back and do nothing can also be enjoyable.

Hallucinations and delusions

at a glance

- Get help from the doctor.
- Explain what is really there if this helps.
- Reassure the person.
- Look for practical solutions such as closing the curtain.
- Explain the situation to others.

Some people with dementia may hear or see things which are not there (hallucinations). This is especially common for people with Lewy body dementia. Some may believe things which are not true (delusions).

More often, people with dementia may mistake what they hear or see for something else, or confuse events. For example, someone may mistake a reflection in the window for someone in the room. Or someone may think things have been stolen because she has forgotten putting them away. These may not be true hallucinations or delusions, but they can still be upsetting or frightening, and the person will need reassurance.

What you can do

1. If the person starts to get hallucinations, make sure she sees the doctor. The problem may be caused by an infection which can be treated. Or it may be a side effect of medicines. Or the doctor may be able to prescribe medicines to stop the hallucinations.

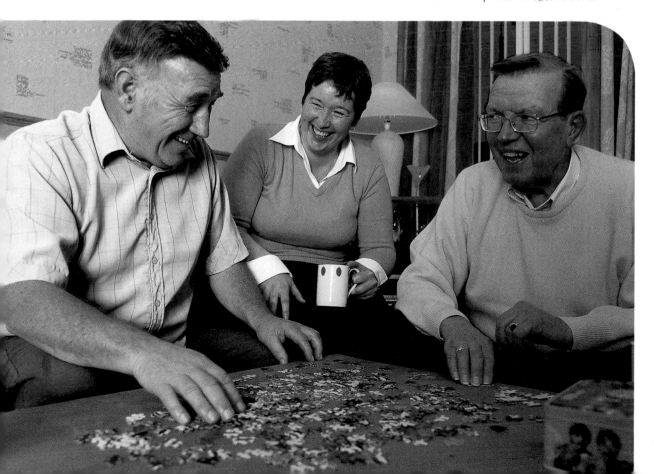

2. If the person misunderstands what she sees, try explaining what it really is. Or change the source of the problem. There may be a simple solution. For example, turn on a light or close the curtains.

3. If the person is really hallucinating, she is experiencing something which is not there. It is pointless to tell her she is imagining it, because it is real to her. Be sympathetic and reassuring. Explain that you cannot see or hear what she can, but that you understand how she feels. Touch and comfort the person in a calm and reassuring way. This may help bring her back to reality.

4. If the person thinks someone is stealing, first check whether this is true. It may not be a delusion – just because someone has dementia does not necessarily mean she is mistaken. Someone who lives alone may be very vulnerable to people who take advantage. If you are sure that the person is deluded, talk to children, home support workers and anyone else who she may accuse of stealing.

Depression and anxiety

at a glance

- **Make sure the person sees her doctor if she seems anxious or depressed.**
- **Be reassuring if the person seems anxious.**
- **Keeping to a routine may help her.**
- **Be positive.**

People with dementia may suffer from anxiety or depression. Anxiety is more common earlier in the illness, when the person is more aware that something is wrong. The person may seem agitated and keep asking the same questions.

Someone may become depressed because the dementia is causing problems like isolation and difficulty in coping. The side effects of drug treatments, physical illness and tiredness can also have an effect.

Because the symptoms of depression and dementia can be similar, it can be hard to know if someone with dementia is depressed. But you might notice her becoming more withdrawn, not sleeping well, lacking energy and interest in things, being more emotional or confused than usual or seeming sad.

What you can do

1. Both depression and anxiety can be treated, so it is important the person sees her doctor.

2. Reassure her if she seems anxious – see **Repeated questions** on page 47.

3. A regular routine can help someone feel more secure.

4. Some people will enjoy stimulating and social activities, but other people may at times feel overwhelmed. Try different things and see what she enjoys.

5. Doing things she enjoys is worthwhile, even if she doesn't remember them afterwards.

6. Say positive things to the person as often as you can.

7. Try to do any important tasks at times of day when the person feels at her best.

Behaviour

Many carers find changes in the behaviour of the person they care for very difficult to handle. But there are a few basic ideas which may help. The person is more likely to feel better in a familiar environment. Try to help her feel secure. If she does something that bothers you, start by thinking about whether it is really a problem. What would happen if she did it again? Perhaps it is risky, or embarrassing. Or perhaps it is just out of the ordinary, but not harmful.

If it is a problem, you may be able to work out what is causing the behaviour. Perhaps you can avoid what starts the behaviour. If you feel there is a problem, always talk to someone about it.

The next few pages cover some of the common difficulties faced by people with dementia and their carers, and some possible solutions. No solution will work for everyone. Try different things until you find what works best.

> *When he has gone to a nearby shop, and not come back, I have to go out searching. I keep my cool when I find him. Sometimes he smiles and says 'I'm glad to see you. I've had a long walk'. Other times he might refuse to get into the car so I let him go. But I keep him in sight until he's tired and agrees to take a lift home.*

'Wandering'

at a glance

- Don't try to prevent 'wandering' if there is no real risk.
- Keep a current photograph.
- Make sure the person gets exercise.
- You may have to stop her from going out alone.
- Give the person identification such as a card, bracelet or pendant.
- If the person is lost, tell the police at once.
- Go along for a walk too and try distraction.
- Make sure she is comfortable and warm at night and reassure her.
- Try to make the house as safe as possible.
- Ask about equipment and services.
- Ask the doctor for a specialist assessment.

Many carers worry about people with dementia 'wandering'. But remember, just because the person may not be able to tell you what she is doing doesn't mean that she is wandering aimlessly. For example, she may be looking for the toilet, feel the need for exercise or have another perfectly good reason for walking about.

If you are worried about the person you care for, ask yourself first whether there is really a problem. If the person goes out, does she find the way home again? Is she able to cross the road safely? Perhaps the person is at risk if she goes out at night but not during the day? Is it a problem if she walks around the house restlessly? Perhaps walking around the house is no problem but going out is a worry.

It is important to give the person as much freedom as reasonably possible – even the freedom to take a risk sometimes.

If the person's walking is a problem, think about why the person is doing it. Is she:

- bored and needing stimulation?

- setting off to do something but forgetting where she was going?

- just going for a walk, perhaps as she has always done?

- unsettled by being in a new and unfamiliar place or finding a familiar place strange?

- needing exercise?

  If the person goes out at night, is she:

- mixed up about the time, not knowing whether it is day or night?

- waking up confused or frightened, not sure where she is?

- looking for the toilet but not able to find it?

- sleeping too much in the day-time or going to bed too early?

- in discomfort or pain for any reason?

- Call the Dementia Helpline for more information – see **Further information** (page 104).

> *My sister used to go out at all hours. I was worried because she's forgotten how to cross the road safely. I put a big notice on the inside of the door to remind her not to go out on her own, and it seems to work most times.*

What you can do

1. Make sure the person gets enough exercise. Try exercise to music or going out for a walk together.

2. Keep a current photograph of the person in case she gets lost.

3. If the person is likely to get lost or be at risk outside, you may have to stop her from going out alone. Try fixing a bell to the door (like a shop door bell) or wind-chimes or an alarm pad under the mat to alert you if she tries to go out. Locking or bolting the house door to stop her going out is dangerous if she is in the house alone. If she is never at home alone, a bolt at the bottom of the outside door where she may not look could stop her going out by herself. But not being able to open the door can make some people with dementia panic.

4. If the person tends to get lost, see that she has identification such as a card, bracelet or pendant. It should show her name and a contact phone number. For security reasons, do not put her address on it. Ask the Dementia Helpline (0808 808 3000) for a Helpcard, which the person can carry and show to someone if she gets confused. The Helpcard also has a space for contact details for emergencies.

5. If the person is lost, tell the police at once. It may help to let them know in advance if she is at risk of getting lost, and giving them a photograph of her.

Day-time

1. Try to find activities which will hold the person's interest. 'Wandering' is less likely if she has something to do.

2. If the person enjoys going for a walk, it is important she can. If she is not safe alone and you can't go along, ask friends or volunteer helpers.

3. If the person with dementia insists on going to see someone who is no longer alive, it is sometimes a good idea to go along too. Gradually divert her attention to things you see or some other topic. Then suggest that it is time to go home. The person may have forgotten the reason for the outing.

Night-time

1. If the person is restless or wants to go out at night, it may help if you increase day-time activity and discourage long sleeps during the day.

2. Make sure that the person has been to the toilet before going to bed.

3. If the person with dementia is restless, make sure she is comfortable and warm. Reassure her about where she is.

4. Leave a dim light on in the bedroom or passage to reduce confusion if the person wakes up in the dark.

5. Try to make the house as safe as possible so that you don't have to worry about the person walking around at night. For example, the occupational therapist may be able to provide an adult stair gate. Lock the kitchen door at night. Put on safe background heating.

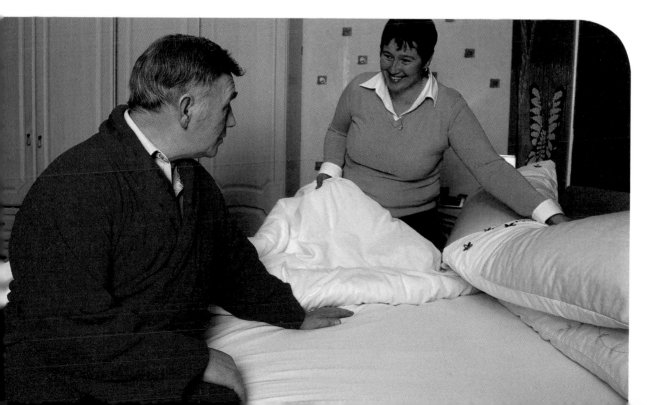

6. The occupational therapist may be able to suggest other equipment to help, such as an alarm pad which will tell you if the person gets out of bed.

7. In some areas a night care service may be available. Call the Dementia Helpline for information, or check with your social work department, Crossroads Caring Scotland or Alzheimer Scotland. In certain circumstances the night nursing service may help – ask the doctor about this.

8. If the person keeps going out and is not safe, ask the doctor for a specialist assessment. Occasionally medication may help but it should not be the doctor's first thought.

Needing attention

at a glance

- Reassure the person.
- Arrange for breaks.

Some people with dementia want to be with their carer all the time. Someone with dementia may follow her carer from room to room, and get very distressed if the carer goes out. This may be very hard for you to bear, especially if it reaches the point where you have no privacy.

The person with dementia may be feeling very insecure. If you leave the room, she may forget where you are or how long you have been away, so she may try to stay with you all the time.

There were times when I found it very hard indeed. She would follow me around everywhere, driving my patience to its limits. My only escape was to lock myself in the bathroom sometimes to read the paper. But now she goes to the day centre, which she loves, and I get two days a week to myself.

What you can do

1. Remember that the person is feeling insecure, and offer plenty of reassurance.

2. Remember that your well-being is important too. You will find it easier to cope with the person's need for attention if you get some time off.

3. Ask for help from family and friends to spend time with the person to give you a break.

4. Consider a day care or home support service (see **Getting help, page 77**) to give you time off.

Anger or aggression

at a glance

- Keep calm.
- Try to defuse the situation.
- Distract the person.
- Don't get involved in an argument.
- Work out what triggers angry outbursts, and try to avoid it.
- Focus on successes.
- Talk about aggression problems with someone you trust.
- Tell the doctor.

Some people can feel aggressive at times as a result of their dementia. Verbal abuse is more common than physical aggression. The person may shout or make accusations or threats. It can be quite a shock if a quiet and gentle person starts to be aggressive.

The person may become aggressive because she is frustrated at not being able to do things she used to be able to do. Or she may misunderstand what is going on. For example, she may put something away and forget it altogether, and then think someone else must have stolen it. Sometimes someone with dementia may over-react to something very minor. The part of the brain which would normally control her reaction may be damaged.

Some people with dementia may be aggressive only to their carers. Perhaps this is because the carer is closest to the person. Many people are more polite to strangers than to people they are close to. This may be very hard to cope with.

What you can do

1. Remain calm if you can, though this is easier said than done. Remind yourself that it is not the person's fault, but the illness making her aggressive or angry. Try not to take it personally. The person will probably quickly forget the anger and upset.

One day I said to my Gran in a calm voice, 'Nobody in this house would steal any of your things. You can't help it because your memory isn't good, even though it can be very upsetting to who you accuse'. She agreed and repeated, 'Nobody in our family steals'. Sarah, aged 10

2. Speak calmly and gently, and try to keep a calm and pleasant expression. Perhaps hold the person's hand. Touching someone can be a good way to help some people feel less isolated; but other people may not like it.

3. Remind the person what is going on around her and what will happen next and why. She is less likely to be frightened if she understands what is going on.

4. Focus on the things the person does well rather than on mistakes or failures.

5. Distract the person's attention away from the situation.

6. If the person is gripping you, try not to struggle. Stay calm and try to defuse the situation.

7. Try not to get into an argument or get angry yourself. This will only make things worse.

8. Afterwards, try to work out what caused the upset and see if there is anything you can change. For example, was she frustrated at failing to do something? If so, perhaps you can make the task easier or avoid it altogether. Explain to other people, such as children or home care workers, that the anger or accusations are caused by the illness.

9. Talk to someone you trust, such as a friend, community psychiatric nurse, social worker or the 24-hour Dementia Helpline. Coping with aggression, especially from someone you love, is very stressful.

10. Ask the doctor for a specialist assessment if you are worried.

11. Remember, aggression does not last for ever. Probably the person you care for will change with time and stop being aggressive.

Embarrassing and odd behaviour

at a glance

- Remember that it is the illness causing the person to behave in this way, and explain this to other people.

- Deal with the situation in a matter-of-fact way.

- If the person tends to lose or hide things, put important items in a secure place.

My father sometimes thinks that I'm my mother and climbs into bed with me. The first time it happened I was very upset. I couldn't understand it. But I talked it over with the community psychiatric nurse and felt a bit better. Now when he does it I get out of bed and leave the room and then come back in saying, 'Hello Dad', to remind him who I am without embarrassing him.

Sometimes someone with dementia may do things which are embarrassing to you. The person will not realise that what she is doing is odd. For example, the person may start to use swear words at embarrassing times, or spit or be rude to visitors. She may do things at the wrong time, such as start to undress in public.

I used to get so upset when my sister ate with her fingers in company. I used to try to make her use her fork, and for a while I didn't invite anyone round. But then I thought about it, and I decided that it really didn't do anyone any harm. She wasn't worried, and my friends all said they didn't mind – it was just me being embarrassed. So I decided not to worry about it any more.

Some embarrassing or odd behaviour may happen because the person is confused about where she is or forgets what should be done when. For some people, the illness may damage the part of the brain that controls their inhibitions, so that they just don't realise that they should not swear in company, for example. Some things the person does may be irritating rather than embarrassing. For example, she may fidget or start to hide things.

Try to think about whether the behaviour really matters, and if so, why. Sometimes you might just be able to learn to live with it.

What you can do

1. Explain what is happening to other people. They will usually be understanding.

2. Don't over-react. For example, if the person starts to undress in company, calmly take her to another room. Make sure that her clothes are comfortable. Check that she is not too hot or wanting to use the toilet.

3. If the person fidgets, try finding her something to do, or just try to ignore the habit. If she fidgets with clothes, try giving her a handkerchief instead.

4. If the person hides things, put important items in a safe place. In time you will get used to where she puts things. It may be a good idea to remove keys from drawers and cupboards.

5. Remember, it is the illness causing the odd behaviour, not the person doing it on purpose.

Sex and intimacy

at a glance

- The person's attitude to sex and intimacy, and her behaviour, may change because of the dementia.
- Discuss problems with someone you trust.
- If you can, give the person plenty of physical contact such as hugs and cuddles.

The person's attitude to sex and sexual relationships may change. People with dementia may sometimes lose interest in sex altogether, or want sex more often than before.

If you are caring for your partner, you may feel differently about sex too. Your relationship may have changed now that you are a carer. You may find that dressing and toileting your partner make it hard to have sexual feelings too. Your partner's personality may have changed.

You may want to carry on your sexual relationship but worry about whether you should. Some partners who continue with a sexual relationship worry that they are taking advantage of the person with dementia. You can usually tell from the person's behaviour whether this is so. Continuing a sexual relationship may help both partners feel closer.

Sometimes someone with dementia may make a sexual approach to someone who is not his or her partner. This might be because the illness has damaged the part of the brain which controls inhibitions.

Or the person might have mistaken someone for his or her partner. Or it may just be that the person wants the comfort of touch and closeness.

Any changes to do with sexual behaviour can be confusing and hard to accept. Sex and relationships can be difficult to talk about, but try to discuss the situation with a professional you trust. Or you can call the Dementia Helpline confidentially and anonymously on **0808 808 3000.** They can send you a free information sheet about sexuality and dementia.

What you can do

1. If you can, give the person plenty of physical contact. Hold hands, or give a hug or a cuddle.

2. If the person approaches the wrong person sexually, stay calm and try to distract and reassure him or her. Remember this is caused by the illness and is not the person's fault.

3. Talk to someone about any problems. Your doctor, local marriage counselling service or Alzheimer Scotland contact may be able to help, or be able to put you in touch with someone who can. They will not be surprised or shocked. Call the 24-hour Dementia Helpline to talk it over confidentially. You don't need to give your name.

> *My wife and I had a very close physical relationship, but since she was diagnosed about four years ago she has gradually lost interest. It bothered me a lot at first, but we still share a bed and that helps me feel close to her. It's something I have come to accept.*

Risks and hazards

Safety in the home

at a glance

- Check for risks and make repairs as needed.
- Fit smoke alarms.
- Make sure lights are bright enough.
- Use fire guards.
- Keep bleach, paints and so on out of reach.
- Make sure that the person can use heaters and cookers safely.
- Ask for advice from the gas supplier.
- Remember that you can't prevent all risks. The person needs freedom too.
- Ask an occupational therapist about safety.

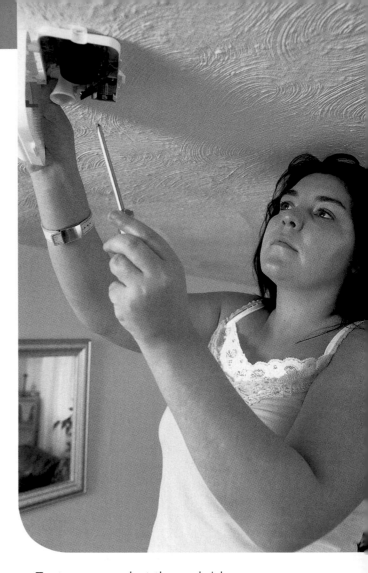

Dementia increases the chance of accidents. It is hard for carers to know how far they should go in trying to protect the person with dementia (or others) from possible risks. It is worth taking a few simple steps to prevent accidents. But you cannot remove all dangers. You can't avoid a certain degree of risk if the person is to keep some independence. If you don't live with the person you care for, safety can be a particular worry.

Try to assess what the real risks are. Observe what the person can and can't do. For example, can she use a gas fire safely? If there is a danger, such as a burning pan, does she react appropriately or not? The booklet *Keeping Safe: A guide to safety when someone with dementia lives alone* gives more information on risk and safety – see **Further information** on page 109. Ask an occupational therapist for help if you are worried.

What you can do

1. Check the home for anything which might cause a fall. Repair or secure any loose banister rails, slippery floor mats and loose carpet edges. Check for badly placed furniture.

2. Electrical appliances and plugs need to be checked regularly. Make sure that cables and wires do not trail across floors. If the person is incontinent don't let her use an electric blanket.

3. Check that bright enough lights are used throughout the house. Use electric night lights to help the person find the way about at night.

4. Fit smoke alarms and make sure neighbours know they are there.

5. The lighting of steps and stairs is very important. You can paint the edge of outside steps with a white line to make it easily seen. An extra hand rail on the stairs can be very helpful.

6. Have hand rails fitted on the bath and by the toilet and put a non-slip mat in the bath or shower.

7. Use a guard in front of any fire. The large 'nursery' type is best, hooked on to the wall or fireplace.

8. Get gas appliances checked for leaks. Your gas company should be able to help – for example, British Gas has a Gas Care Register for people who are disabled or over 60 and living alone or with other people over 60. This gives the right to a free safety check every year.

9. Keep cleaning fluids, bleach, paints and so on out of reach. Some people with dementia may mistake them for ordinary drinks.

10. If the person cooks or lights a fire, make sure she can still do this safely. Put large clear instructions beside the appliance. If the person cannot use appliances safely make sure that she only uses them when someone is there. Using only one gas ring lessens the danger. Your gas company can arrange this. An automatic electric kettle may be useful if the person can learn to use it.

11. If the person becomes unsafe with a gas fire, it may be better replaced. Some carers recommend an oil-filled electric radiator or an electric heater on a timer switch.

12. Ask an occupational therapist for help. He or she should be able to tell you about aids and equipment such as devices to turn off taps if they are left on.

13. Ask the social work department about alarm systems. In some areas systems are available which can help someone who lives alone even if she can't sound an alarm herself. For example, they might alert someone if a tap is left running, or if the person doesn't get out of bed at her usual time.

> *My father's neighbour was worried about him using his gas cooker because a couple of times he forgot to light it. But he didn't want to stop cooking. I talked to the gas board, who fitted a gas isolation tap. Now he cooks his lunch while his home help is there to help him, and she turns the gas off when she leaves.*

Driving

at a glance

- Ask the doctor if the person is safe to drive.
- Tell the insurance company and the DVLA of the person's diagnosis.
- Discuss with the person with dementia when driving should stop.
- Consider other ways to travel.

> *My mother used to rely on her car and didn't want to stop driving. But I could see that she wasn't safe any more. In the end it was the doctor who told her she'd have to stop. He said she should think of it as if she was finding it hard to see properly.*

> *I tried to get my husband to stop driving but he just wouldn't be told. I was worried in the car with him. I had to remind him which way to go round roundabouts. I hid the car keys but he got angry and threatened me. In the end my son took a vital bit out of the engine, so the car wouldn't start. He was frustrated for a while but at least he didn't blame me.*

Generally people with moderate to severe dementia will not be able to drive. However, some people early on in the illness may continue to drive safely for a while. If you are not sure if the person is safe to drive, and she still wants to, her doctor can refer her to the Scottish Driving Assessment Service to check if she is still safe to drive. You must tell the insurance company and the DVLA about a diagnosis of dementia.

If the person is not safe to drive, discuss it with her – she may be ready to give up. It is a difficult issue but don't wait until there is an accident. If you can't persuade her to stop, contact the DVLA. They will check with her doctor and if necessary they can take away her licence.

Call the Dementia Helpline for an information sheet about driving and dementia.

What you can do

1. Encourage the person to get used to other transport such as buses and trains.

2. Raise the subject of driving tactfully. Point out the hazards. If possible, also point out the benefits of not having to drive.

3. If the person does not want to stop driving, ask other carers how they handled the problem.

4. The person may find it easier to accept that she must stop driving if someone in authority says so. Ask the doctor or the police to help.

5. Make other arrangements for transport. Try to make up a rota of drivers or suggest using buses. Some groups such as the WRVS may be able to help with transport. Check with the social work department, as some local councils have taxi schemes for disabled people.

Smoking and alcohol

at a glance

- Try to persuade the person with dementia to stop smoking.
- Keep matches out of reach.
- Put big ashtrays everywhere.
- Fit smoke alarms.
- Don't leave alcohol where the person can drink unsupervised.
- Ask the doctor whether the person should drink alcohol.

Smoking and drinking cause problems in dementia. Smoking is a fire hazard for people who are forgetful. A drink or two causes slight loss of mental alertness in anyone. For a person with dementia such a loss has greater effects and could increase confusion. The occasional drink in company is not always a bad idea. However, care and supervision are needed. There may be extra risks when someone is on medication and has a drink.

What you can do

1. Try to persuade the person with dementia to stop smoking or cut down. Many people with dementia forget to smoke and then do not miss the habit once it is broken.

2. Some people smoke more when they are bored, so try to make sure the person has plenty of company and stimulation.

3. Make sure she does not abandon lighted cigarettes or throw them away in wastepaper baskets. Stop the person from smoking in bed if you can.

4. Put big ashtrays everywhere. Put an ashtray at hand height beside the person's favourite chair. Replace wastepaper baskets with metal bins.

5. Fit smoke alarms in all rooms. A heat detector might be more suitable in the bedroom, if there is a risk that the person may smoke in bed, because it goes off sooner if there is a fire.

6. Keep matches out of reach.

7. Buy flame-resistant clothes and furniture.

8. If the person is using nicotine patches make sure she does not smoke, as this greatly increases the health risks.

9. Don't leave alcohol where the person with dementia can help herself. The person may not remember how much she has had. You may have to lock alcohol up or hide it.

10. Ask the doctor's advice about whether the person can have any alcoholic drink and, if so, how much. This is essential if the person is taking medicines.

> *My brother has always liked a few drinks, but he started forgetting how many he'd had and drinking far too much. My sister and I do his shopping now, so we bought some low alcohol lager to see if he'd like it. He still gets through a lot of cans – but at least he doesn't get drunk now.*

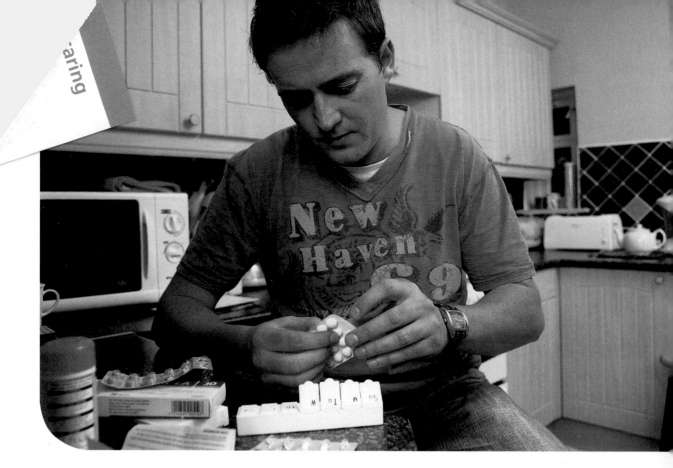

Medicines

at a glance

- Ask the doctor if medicines are necessary and if they can be given as simply as possible.

- Don't leave the person to take medicines alone.

- Work out a system for making sure that the person takes the right medicine at the right time.

- Watch for side effects and inform the doctor.

- Make sure that the doctor knows about all medicines the person is taking.

- Get rid of medicines not in use.

You will have to take special care if the person with dementia is on any sort of medicine. She may forget how many tablets she has had. She may accidentally take too many or not take them at all. Check with the doctor to make sure the person is only taking what is necessary.

What you can do

1. Ask the doctor if each medicine is really necessary. If it is, ask if the person can take it in a simpler way, such as once a day instead of three times.

2. Do not leave it to the person with dementia to see to medication. She is likely to forget or to take too much. It is better if one person is in charge of medicines.

3. If you can't supervise medication completely, there are several ideas which might help.

You can leave the right daily dose in containers. Ask the pharmacist about special containers with compartments for each dose. You can also get dispensers with an alarm, or which you can set to open at a certain time.

4. Keep all medicine bottles clearly labelled and in a locked medicine cupboard.

5. Keep a weekly or monthly record sheet on the inside of the medicine cupboard. Note on the sheet which tablets the person should take each day. When you give a tablet, mark the record sheet to show that you have given it. This helps to stop mistakes, especially if more than one person is involved.

6. Make sure that you are clear about which medicine to give when. If not, check with the doctor or pharmacist.

7. Make sure that both the hospital doctor and the GP know about all the drugs the person is taking. Even medicines bought over the counter, such as laxatives or aspirin, can cause problems when taken with other medicines.

8. Make a note of any side effects and let the doctor know.

9. Get rid of medicines not in use.

> *When I looked in my father-in-law's medicine cabinet I found almost twenty different prescription drugs. Some dated back more than five years. I checked with his doctor and he was only on one pill three times a day. So I took the rest to the chemist's to be disposed of.*

getting help

The national 24-hour Dementia Helpline on **0808 808 3000** is a good place to start. They can help you work out what help might be useful and can put you in touch with local services near you. There are free guides to local services for people with dementia and their carers for many parts of Scotland. Ask the Dementia Helpline if there is one for your area.

Community care services

at a glance

- The social work department arranges community care and carers' assessments.

- The person with dementia has a right to a community care assessment.

- You have a right to a carer's assessment.

- Home care services (sometimes called domiciliary services) support the person at home.

- Day centres are enjoyable for the person and give you a break.

- Respite breaks can give you some time to yourself.

- You and the person may benefit from a holiday.

- The social work department can arrange services such as laundry or meals.

- If you are not satisfied you can ask for a review or make a complaint.

The person with dementia has a right to a **community care assessment.**

Call your local social work department to ask for this. They will arrange for a social worker or another community care professional to visit and talk to you and the person with dementia. Increasingly, in some areas, a health care professional such as a community psychiatric nurse or a voluntary sector worker may be able to do the assessment. It is often a good idea to spend some time talking in private with the person doing the assessment, so that you feel more able to be open about anything that you are concerned about. He or she will probably also talk to other people with relevant information, such as the doctor.

> *My mother is very good at being polite and sociable. She thinks she does all her own cooking and shopping, but in fact I do everything. But she gets very anxious and confused when I'm not with her. When the social worker came to assess my mother I was worried he wouldn't see the true picture. So I asked him to stay with my other for ten minutes while I nipped out to the shops. When I came back he said, 'I don't know how you've been coping'.*

Separately from that, you, as the carer, have a right to a **carer's assessment** if you are providing 'substantial and regular' care – which most carers of people with dementia will be. The social work department, health service and any other organisation involved in providing services should treat you

77

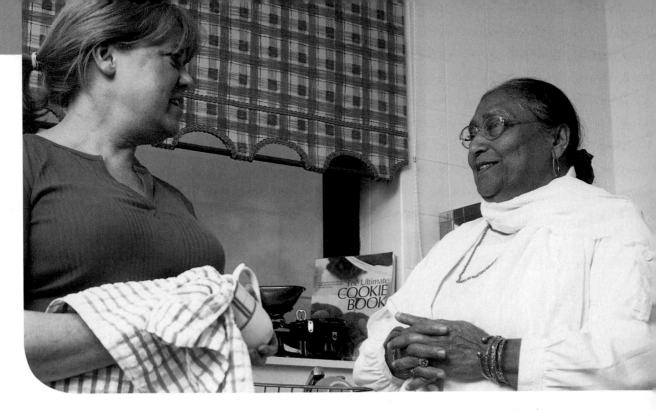

as a 'key partner' in providing care to the person with dementia. They should use the special knowledge you have of the person to make sure that she gets the services that are right for her. They should give you support and advice. They should also provide care services to the person that will support you to care for her as much as and for as long as you want to, and feel able to.

If the assessment shows that the person with dementia needs services, the person doing the assessment will put together a **care plan.** They should give the person a copy. The care plan will set out details of a 'package of care', using local services to try to meet the needs of the person with dementia. Services may be provided by the social work department or by voluntary or private organisations. Assessment is free, but you may have to pay for some services (see **Free personal care and charges for care services,** page 82).

Sometimes there is a waiting list for assessments. If you need help right away, ask the social work department if they can do an emergency assessment.

The social work department must also provide aftercare services to people with dementia leaving hospital. One month's care in the person's own home is free, including non-personal care.

Help at home

Home care services (sometimes called domiciliary services) can offer care for the person with dementia in her own home, depending on what she needs. For example, a home help might help the person to prepare a meal, or a care assistant might help her to get dressed or go out for a walk. For many carers, this gives the freedom of a few hours without worry. Home care services can also help people with dementia who live alone to cope and to live at home safely for as long as possible. In some areas, overnight home care services may be available to enable a carer to get a good night's sleep. Ask the social work department or call the Dementia Helpline for details of services in your area.

Home help

Home helps, also known in different areas as home carers or home care assistants, are provided by the social work department. In many areas, home helps are now providing personal care services more than, for example, doing the cleaning. Often they also provide much-needed company.

Home support services

Some voluntary organisations provide home support or 'sitter' services. For example, Crossroads and Alzheimer Scotland run schemes in many areas, providing trained care assistants to help look after the person with dementia. They do more than just 'sit' with the person. They can provide stimulating activities or outings, for example.

Private nursing or care agencies can also provide care assistants or nurses during the day or at night. You can find them in the local Yellow Pages.

> *My husband didn't want to go to the day centre at all. Although he's 81, he hated the idea of 'sitting around with all those old people'. But I persuaded him to try it and went with him the first couple of times and now he loves it. They go on outings, and he gets a game of snooker with one of the volunteers most days. Now he goes twice a week and I get the peace and quiet I need to help me cope.*

Day centres

A place at a day centre can give the person with dementia a chance to socialise and to enjoy stimulating activities. It will also give you some time off. Most day centres will arrange transport. Evening and weekend care is also available in some areas. Some day centres are run by the social work department, others by voluntary organisations such as Alzheimer Scotland.

Specialist day centres provide activities suited to the person's abilities. They can often cater even for people whose dementia is quite severe.

In some areas there are now day centres particularly for younger people with dementia. But in many areas younger people go to day centres which cater mostly for older people. If you care for a younger person, ask the social work department about services in your area.

Respite breaks

Everyone needs time off sometimes. Caring for someone with dementia can be a tiring and often stressful job. A respite break, when the person with dementia goes into a care home, or sometimes a hospital for a few days or a week or two, will give you the chance to recharge your batteries. Perhaps you might take a holiday, or maybe just have some time for yourself at home. Don't feel you have to visit the person – this is a time to give yourself a break. Perhaps family and friends could visit rather than you. In some areas social work or health professionals can arrange a programme of regular respite breaks for you.

There are three routes to respite.

Respite through the social work department

If you are assessed as needing respite, the social worker or care manager should try to arrange a place in a care home for the person. If you haven't been assessed as needing respite, but you feel you need a break, call the social work department and ask for a new assessment. There may be a charge for respite care. The amount depends on where you live and on the person's income and capital.

Respite through the health service

In some areas, the GP or hospital specialist can sometimes arrange a respite place in hospital. There is no charge for this.

> *I felt very guilty about letting my father go into respite care for a fortnight. Last time he went he came back more confused because of the change of environment, although the home said he was fine while he was there. But when I talked it over at the carers' group they pointed out that I must look after myself if I want to go on looking after him for as long as I can. And he settled down again after a few days.*

Private respite

If you arrange respite in a care home privately, you will have to pay the home's fees. Make sure the home you choose is suitable. Visit, preferably with the person you care for, talk to the staff and, if you can, talk to residents and their relatives.

Meals services

Meals on Wheels and other similar services can provide hot meals or in some areas frozen meals, delivered to the person's house. Ask the social work department about the service.

Holidays

Both you and the person with dementia may enjoy a holiday, either together or separately. Many people with dementia manage very well in hotels or guest houses, but for information on other places which are suitable for people with dementia, call the Dementia Helpline.

Laundry service

Some areas have a laundry service for people who have extra washing because of continence problems. Ask the social work department or the community nurse.

If the person does not want the service

Someone with dementia may not want to accept a service for a number of reasons. Perhaps the person thinks she is coping perfectly well, and doesn't realise the need for help. Perhaps she is reluctant to have a stranger in the house. Or she may have negative ideas about day centres. She may not want to go into respite care for fear of being taken away from home. Often this is more of a problem earlier in the illness, when the person may feel that independence is being taken away. Later, she may be less unwilling.

Even when someone is initially unwilling to accept a service, she is quite likely to enjoy it and benefit from it once she starts. So it is worth persisting.

What you can do

1. Talk to the person with dementia about the service you think might help. Try to explain why you think it is a good idea, and how the service will help both of you.

2. Talk to the social worker, nurse or someone else for advice.

3. Suggest a trial period. The person may well find that she enjoys a day centre, for example.

4. Try going with the person to a day centre for the first few visits, or being there when a home care worker comes.

5. Reassure her that respite is just for a holiday and that she will be coming home.

If you are not satisfied

The social work department will usually try to provide a service. But sometimes you may not agree with what they think you and the person need. Or you may be told the person can't have a service because there is no space, or because the social work department does not have the money. If you are not satisfied, ask for a review of the assessment or the care plan. The social work department should look at it again and may agree to make changes.

If you are still not satisfied, make a complaint. There is no right of appeal in community care law. But every social work department must by law have a complaints procedure. Ask them for information on how to make a complaint. You can get help with making a complaint from the Dementia Helpline.

> *My wife hated the idea of going into respite and I put it off for a long time. But I was making myself ill, getting up with her two or three times a night. Eventually I told her that I needed the break and she agreed to go just for the weekend. When she came back from the home she wanted to know how soon she could go back to 'that lovely hotel'!*

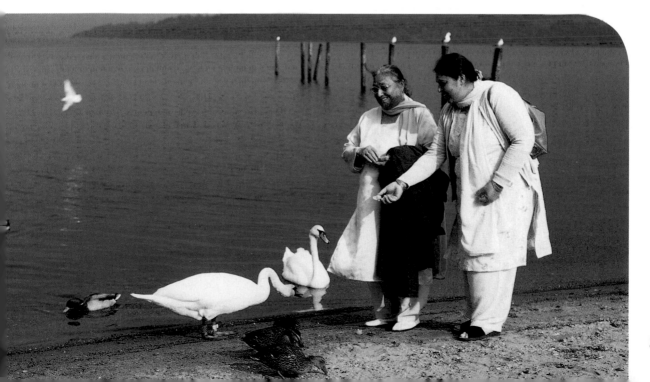

You can make comments to the social work department as well as complaints. You may wish to point out gaps in services which you feel should be given priority.

Free personal care and charges for care services

at a glance

- People over 65 can get free personal care at home.
- Nursing care at home is free for people of any age.
- The person may have to pay for some other services.

Free personal care

If the person with dementia is over 65, and she is assessed as needing help at home with personal care, she will not have to pay for this help. However, people under 65 still have to pay. Personal care includes, for example, help with dressing, eating, washing, going to the toilet, simple treatments such as eye drops, staying safe and support such as reminders. Someone can get free personal care whatever their income and savings.

Nursing care at home is free, whatever the person's age.

Charges for care services

Whether or not the person gets free personal care, she may still have to pay for some services, such as day care, lunch clubs, meals on wheels, community alarms, help with shopping and housework or respite breaks. Each social work department has different charges for services. The social worker or care manager will do a financial assessment to work out how much someone can afford to pay. The amount depends on the income and individual circumstances of the person with dementia. Many people pay nothing at all or only a small amount.

Direct payments

at a glance

- People with dementia can get direct payments.
- You can manage direct payments for someone if you are her attorney or guardian.
- Direct payments mean you can choose and pay for services that meet the person's needs, or employ someone to provide care.

If the assessment shows that the person with dementia needs community care services, the social work department must offer the option of direct payments. Direct payments mean that instead of the social work department organising the services, the person can be given the money to arrange and pay for services. People with moderate to severe dementia would usually need someone else to manage this for them. You can do this if you have power of attorney for the person, or have been appointed her guardian (see **Money and legal matters,** page 28).

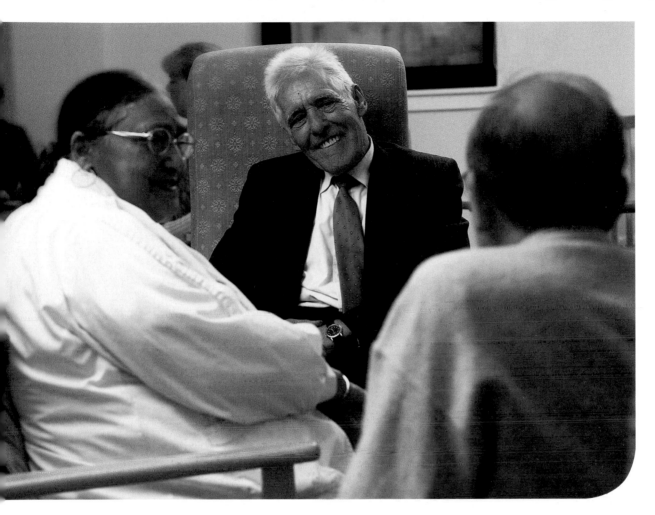

If you get direct payments you must spend the money on meeting those needs. You can't spend it on anything else. You can either buy services from private or voluntary providers, or employ someone to provide the care.

Direct payments can give you more control and choice over exactly what services are provided and when. You can also choose to have a mixture of direct payments and services.

If you think you might want direct payments, ask the social work department for more information.

Health services for people with dementia

at a glance

- See the GP if you have any concerns about the person's health.

- It is especially important that the person sees the GP if there is a sudden change in her health.

- The GP can refer the person to hospital specialists and other health services.

- The person can get an assessment at a hospital assessment unit or day hospital.

- If you are not satisfied, you can talk to the doctor, change doctor or make a complaint.

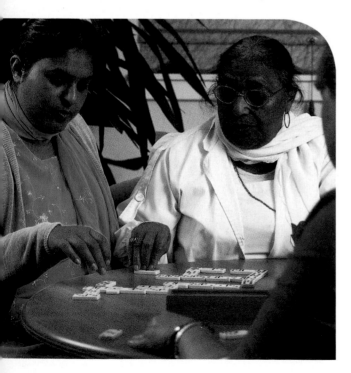

Seeing the doctor

If you are concerned about the health, physical or mental, of the person you care for, you can talk to her family doctor or general practitioner (GP). Make an appointment. If you have a lot to discuss, ask for a double appointment or a time at the end of a surgery so that you don't feel rushed. Make a list before you go so that you remember everything you want to say.

It is important to tell the doctor at once if there is a sudden change. Don't just assume that any change is due to dementia. For example, if the person suddenly seems more confused she may have an infection. If this is treated, the confusion may get better.

If you can, talk to the person you care for before visiting the doctor. If the person agrees, you can be with her when she sees the doctor. Early on in the illness, the doctor may not be able to tell you about the person's health without her permission because of confidentiality. But your information will help the doctor, especially when the person does not have a clear idea of her own problems. Later, the doctor will probably feel it is in the person's best interest to discuss her health with you, as her carer.

The GP may refer the person to a hospital specialist or a memory clinic for diagnosis or treatment. The GP or specialist can also arrange for other health services such as a day hospital or an assessment in hospital.

Alzheimer Scotland has a useful booklet called *Getting help from your doctor.* Call the Dementia Helpline on **0808 808 3000** for a free copy.

Memory clinics

In some places there are memory clinics, which provide diagnosis, assessment or treatment for people with dementia. Different memory clinics operate in different ways, but they will have specialist doctors and other health professionals. They may also provide information and support with coping with the illness, or refer you to someone else for this.

Day hospital

The person with dementia may be offered a place at a day hospital. At the day hospital, she can be medically assessed. The day hospital may offer services such as occupational therapy assessment, nursing assessment, physiotherapy, bathing or podiatry (chiropody). The person with dementia will be able to take part in stimulating activities. A place at a day hospital for the person you care for will also give you some time for yourself. Day hospitals do not usually offer longer term support. They may refer the person on to a day centre.

> *My mother's care manager found her a place at a day centre for three days and one evening a week, plus a sitter service every Saturday morning and one evening a fortnight. She goes into respite for a week every three months too. It means that I can work part time and get some time with my family, while still caring for her.*

Assessment units

The doctor may arrange for the person to go into an assessment unit in the hospital. The person can be given special diagnostic tests if they are necessary. Or the unit may try to help with a particularly troubling problem such as hallucinations or aggression.

If you are not satisfied with the GP or hospital service

Every part of the National Health Service has a complaints procedure. Ask for information on how to make a complaint.

If you are not satisfied with the GP's diagnosis or with the service he or she gives, you can:

- speak to the GP about it

- see another GP in the practice

- change GP by asking another GP to put you on his or her list – you don't need to tell your GP you're going to do this

- ask for a second opinion from a specialist

- make a complaint.

If you are unhappy with a hospital service, you can:

- speak to the person in charge

- make a complaint.

If you are not happy with the outcome of your complaint, you can ask for an independent review.

Information and support

at a glance

- The 24-hour Dementia Helpline on 0808 808 3000 can provide information and emotional support.
- Try joining a carers' support group.
- Advocacy can help the person with dementia or carer be listened to.
- Your local health promotion department can provide information materials.
- If you are worried what would happen to the person if you were taken ill, carry emergency details.
- Voluntary organisations such as Alzheimer Scotland can provide information and services.

Dementia Helpline

The 24-hour Dementia Helpline is on **0808 808 3000.** Calls are free. The Helpline is answered by trained staff and volunteers, many of whom have been carers themselves. They can give information on anything to do with dementia, from how to cope with particular problems to where to find services locally. They also offer emotional support. You can talk over your feelings or use the Helpline as a shoulder to cry on, day or night, 365 days a year. Your call is confidential and you don't even have to give your name.

Carers' support groups

A carers' support group gives you the chance to meet other people who also care for someone, for emotional support and good ideas and tips on coping. Many carers' support groups also have guest speakers who are a very useful source of information. Some are organised by day care and other services. Ask the Dementia Helpline or the social work department about groups near you.

Courses for carers

Some organisations run courses for carers. Sometimes these are just for carers of people with dementia and sometimes for all carers. Courses may cover different things. Examples of topics included on a course might be information about dementia, how to cope, what help is available, financial and legal matters and dealing with stress. Ask the Dementia Helpline to put you in touch with your nearest Alzheimer Scotland service or a local carers' organisation.

Advocacy

Some areas have independent advocacy services. They offer advice and support for people with dementia who need help to make sure their views are represented. There are also some advocacy services especially for carers. Ask the social work department, the Dementia Helpline or the Scottish Independent Advocacy Alliance (see **Further information** on pages 104 and 106).

Health promotion

Your local health promotion office can provide leaflets, videos and information on local support groups. They can also provide information on conferences. Find them in the 'phone book listed under the health board.

Carer's emergency card

You may be worried about what would happen to the person you look after if you were in an accident or taken ill. If so, carry a note of who to contact in an emergency. Some carer organisations provide a special card you can fill in with details of who you care for and emergency contacts. Call the Dementia Helpline if you would like one.

Voluntary organisations

Many voluntary organisations can help you care for the person with dementia. Some, like Alzheimer Scotland, Crossroads or Age Concern Scotland, and many small local organisations, may provide services such as day care or home support. They may provide information, someone to talk to or carers' groups. See **Further information** on page 102 for more details on individual voluntary organisations.

The people who help

at a glance

- Social worker.
- Care manager.
- Family doctor.
- Old age psychiatrist.
- Psychiatrist or neurologist.
- Community psychiatric nurse.
- Community nurse.
- Practice nurse.
- Health visitor.
- Occupational therapist.
- Clinical psychologist.
- Podiatrist (chiropodist).
- Dentist.

Different social work departments and health boards organise services in different ways. In some areas staff will work in specialist dementia teams. In some areas, community care assessments are mostly done by social workers. In other areas they may be done by occupational therapists, community psychiatric nurses or other professionals as well as social workers. Increasingly in many areas, health and social work are working more closely together, so the assessment may be done by one member of a team which has several different kinds of professionals (a 'multi-disciplinary team'). The team might also include professionals from specialist voluntary organisations. This section will give you an idea of what each person specialises in.

Social worker

The social worker will often be the person who visits and assesses the needs of the person with dementia and of the carer. He or she should know what services are available locally and help you access services both within the social work department and elsewhere. For example, if the person with dementia needs day care, the social worker will try to find a place at a suitable day centre. Social workers can find you help with problems, both practical and to do with emotions or relationships. They can be a source of advice and support for the family.

Care manager

The care manager might be from social work, the health service or the voluntary sector. He or she may be the person who provides the assessment. The care manager's job is to organise a 'package of care' for someone who needs a lot of help.

Family doctor

The family doctor or general practitioner can be a very good source of help and information. He or she can help make sure the person with dementia stays as physically healthy as possible. He or she can put you in touch with other health professionals such as community nurses, physiotherapists, health visitors and hospital services.

Old age psychiatrist, psychiatrist or neurologist

People who are over 65 and have dementia, or have memory problems but have not been diagnosed may be referred to an old age psychiatrist (or psychogeriatrician) at a local hospital. Old age psychiatrists are doctors who specialise in the physical and mental health needs of older people.

People who are under 65 and have dementia, or have memory problems but have not yet been diagnosed may be referred to a psychiatrist or a neurologist at a local hospital. Psychiatrists are doctors who specialise in mental health, including dementia. Neurologists specialise in illnesses of the brain. In some areas, people under 65 with dementia may be referred to an old age psychiatrist.

If you would like the person you care for to see a specialist, ask the GP to refer her. Patients have a right to a second opinion.

Community psychiatric nurse

Community psychiatric nurses (CPNs) can give emotional support and practical advice to help both carers and people with dementia throughout the illness. They may be able to visit regularly and get to know both you and the person with dementia. This means they are ideally placed to offer support and guidance through the many changes dementia brings. They offer information about the illness and on practical ways of coping. They can help with changes in the person's behaviour, and they can also monitor treatments. They will know what services are available locally and can help you get them. At any stage you can ask your GP to arrange for a CPN to visit.

Community nurse

The community nurse can visit to assess and advise on the nursing needs of the person with dementia, such as bathing or incontinence. Ask the GP or contact the community nursing service directly. In most areas they are based at the health centre or GP surgery.

Practice nurse

The practice nurse is based at the GP surgery and can give help and advice on health problems.

Health visitor

A health visitor can assess and advise on any problems related to health. Contact the health visitor at the health centre or GP surgery.

Occupational therapist

The occupational therapist (OT) is expert at helping people to continue doing as much as they can in their daily lives, for example with social and practical activities. An OT can visit the person at home to assess risks and suggest ways to improve safety, maintain independence and enhance psychological well-being. He or she can recommend the right equipment to help, from bath and toilet aids to memory aids. You might be able to borrow equipment to try it out. You can find an OT through the social work department or through the hospital psychiatric service.

Clinical psychologist

A clinical psychologist can work with people with dementia to help them learn ways of overcoming difficulties or coping better. He or she may be able to help with behavioural changes, such as aggression, 'wandering' and self-care problems.

The clinical psychologist can help carers deal with stress and feelings such as grief.

Clinical psychologists are usually based in hospitals. Ask the GP or a dementia team member if you would like to see a clinical psychologist.

Podiatrist (chiropodist)

Podiatrists (the new name for chiropodists) usually work in clinics, but can make home visits. Most people with dementia will be able to get free podiatry. Ask your doctor or the podiatry department of your local health board for details.

Dentist

Some dentists will do home visits. Talk to the person's dentist about this or ask your local health board about the Community Dental Service.

long-stay care

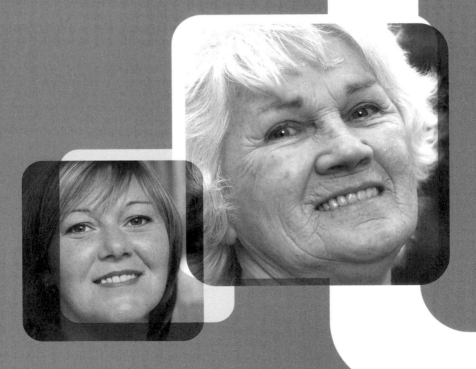

long-stay care

The decision

at a glance

- There may come a time when it is not possible to go on caring at home.
- Involve the person with dementia in the decision as much as you can.
- Involve other people, to share responsibility for the decision.

Eventually, you may not be able to go on looking after the person with dementia at home. Perhaps she has become so ill she needs a team of people to care for her. Or perhaps your own health has changed. Not everyone can be a carer and not everyone can go on caring as long as they wish they could. It is important to understand and accept what you can and can't do. Most people with dementia are likely to need to move into long-stay care in the later stages of their illness.

Try not to take this difficult decision on your own. Involve the person as much as you can, and take into account any wishes she may have expressed in the past. But remember that things change, and sometimes it may be in the person's best interest to move into a home, even if that isn't what she would have hoped for.

Involve other family members too if you can. But if they disagree, remember that as the carer, you know the person and the situation best. Professionals such as the social worker, doctor, nurse or staff at services the person uses can help you. It may help to talk as well to other carers who have had to make a decision about long-stay care.

Alzheimer Scotland has a helpful booklet, *A positive choice: Choosing long-stay care for a person with dementia*. The booklet looks at how to cope with the emotional effects of deciding on long-stay care, and covers the practicalities in detail. Call the Dementia Helpline on **0808 808 3000** for a free copy.

Coping with your feelings

at a glance

- It is normal to have difficult feelings such as guilt.
- Talk to someone about how you are feeling.

It may be very hard for you to accept that you can no longer provide care for the person with dementia. You may feel guilty or think that other people will disapprove. It may be hard to know what you will do with all the spare time you suddenly have. You may feel lonely without the person you were looking after and feel a sense of loss.

It is probably impossible to avoid difficult and painful feelings. It may help to talk to friends or professionals about how you feel, or to call the Dementia Helpline. It can also be helpful to talk to other carers at a carers' support group.

> *Admitting to myself that I couldn't go on looking after my partner was very hard. I now realise I struggled on far too long because I felt so bad about letting other people care for her. But now she's in a nursing home quite nearby and she's getting better care than I could manage on my own. And I feel much more relaxed. I visit her often and because I no longer have to do all the routine tasks I find I enjoy our time together much more.*

In time you will probably realise that your decision is for the best. It can be a comfort to see the person settle in and enjoy your visits. Although the home will cope with the day-to-day caring, you can still be involved. Taking the person out for a walk, a run in the car or a day at home may still be possible. You may also be able to help with personal care, if you want to.

Arranging long-stay care

at a glance

- Get a community care assessment to see what sort of care the person needs.
- Get a carer's assessment for yourself.

The best way to arrange long-stay care is to ask the social work department for a **community care assessment.** An assessment will make sure the person gets the right kind of care to meet her needs. A community care assessment is essential for the person to be able to get the free personal or nursing care allowance towards the home fees. It is also important for her to have an assessment if she needs help paying the fees now, or might need help in the future.

You have a right to a carer's assessment for yourself, too. This will look at how you are coping, and how able you are to go on caring. To do the assessments, a social worker, care manager or another professional will talk to you and to others involved in the person's care.

The assessment may show that moving into a care home is the best option for the person. Or sometimes it may be that there are other services which could help you cope at home for longer, if you want to.

If the person is assessed as needing long-stay care, the local authority can arrange it, or you can choose to arrange it yourself.

Choosing a home

at a glance

- The Care Commission registers and inspects care homes and can give you information about them.
- Visit several homes before you make a choice.

- You can choose a home in another part of the UK.
- You can choose a more expensive home than the local authority will pay for if someone can top up the fees.
- An independent advocate may be helpful.

Most people with dementia who need long-stay care will move into a care home. Care homes may be run by private companies, the social work department or voluntary organisations. Care homes provide different levels of care – for example, some provide nursing care. All care homes have to meet National Care Standards.

All care homes in Scotland are registered and inspected by the Care Commission (see **Further information, page 103**). The Care Commission

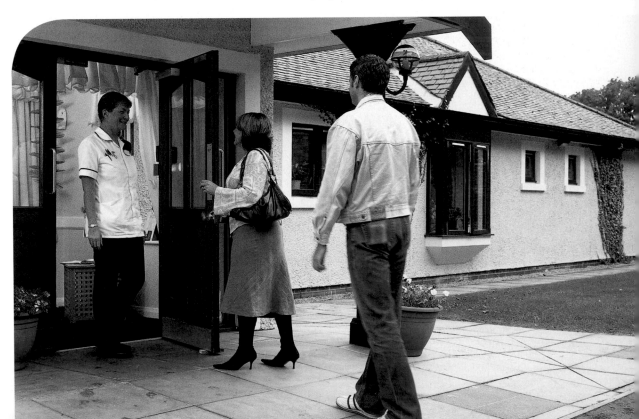

can give you a list of homes in any area, and copies of inspection reports for homes you are considering.

The local authority has a maximum amount they will normally pay for home fees. They should offer the person a place in a home that is suitable and within this maximum. Or they may provide a list of homes for you to choose from. If you can, visit several homes before you decide on which would best suit the person with dementia. Perhaps you and the person can visit together. The booklet *A positive choice* has a useful checklist of what to consider when you visit a home.

You can also choose a different home, anywhere in the UK, as long as it is suitable for the person's needs and doesn't cost more than the local authority normally pays. Or, if it costs more, you or someone else can agree to pay the extra, bearing in mind that, if you stop paying for any reason, the person may have to move.

It may be helpful to involve an independent advocate when you are making these decisions. He or she can represent the wishes of the person with dementia without being emotionally involved. Call the Dementia Helpline or the Scottish Independent Advocacy Alliance (see **Further information** on pages 104 and 106) to find out about advocacy services near you.

A few people with dementia who have very complex needs may need continuing NHS care. This decision is up to the person's consultant.

Paying the home fees

at a glance

- People over 65 paying all or part of their own fees can get free personal care.
- People of any age paying all or part of their own fees can get free nursing care.
- The social work department will do a financial assessment to see how much the person should pay towards her fees.
- The value of the person's house will be counted in some circumstances but not in others.

Free personal care

In Scotland, anyone living in a care home who is over 65 and paying some or all of the fees is entitled to free personal care (as long as he or she is assessed as needing personal care). Nursing care in care homes is free for people of any age who are assessed as needing it.

The local authority pays the allowance for free personal care or free nursing care, or both, direct to the home. The person then pays the rest of the fees, which are for food, accommodation and so on.

From 1 April 2008 the amount for personal care is £169 per week, and for nursing care it is £67 per week.

Other help towards the fees

Care home fees can be hundreds of pounds a week. Many people will need some help with paying. The social work department will give the person a financial assessment. They will look at the person's income and capital. The person's income will be used to pay the home fees. She should always be left with a weekly personal allowance (at least £21.15 from April 2008, plus up to £5.45 more for some people over 65 receiving Pension Credit, depending on savings and income).

If the person's income is not enough to pay the full fees, the local authority may help to pay the amount over her income. If the person has savings or property worth more than the 'upper limit' (£21,500 from April 2008), she will have to pay the home fees herself until the amount reduces to this level. If she has an amount between the upper limit and the 'lower limit' (£13,000 from April 2008), she will have to pay part of the fees and the local authority will pay part. If she has less than the lower limit, the social work department will pay, up to their maximum amount.

The house

If the person owns a house the social work department will normally count it as part of her capital if she moves into a care home permanently. They can count its value, less any mortgage and less 10% of the house's value to cover selling costs. But they must ignore the value of the house for the first 12 weeks of the person's stay in the care home.

However, the social work department must ignore the value of the house completely if one of these people still lives there:

- person's husband or wife, or opposite sex partner

- a relative who is over 60

- a relative who is disabled or incapacitated.

The social work department can also decide to ignore the value of the house if someone else still lives there, such as a carer or a same-sex partner. Seek advice from the Dementia Helpline or a solicitor if you live with the person with dementia and the social work department say they will take the house into account.

The move and after

at a glance

- Plan the move.
- Personalise the person's room with familiar things.
- Talk to the home about how she is settling in, and about her care plan.
- Give it time – both you and the person with dementia will need to adjust.
- If you're not happy about the person's care, talk to the home first, and make a complaint if you are still not satisfied.

Spending time planning before the person moves can help to make it easier for both of you. You will have to cope with practical issues as well as with

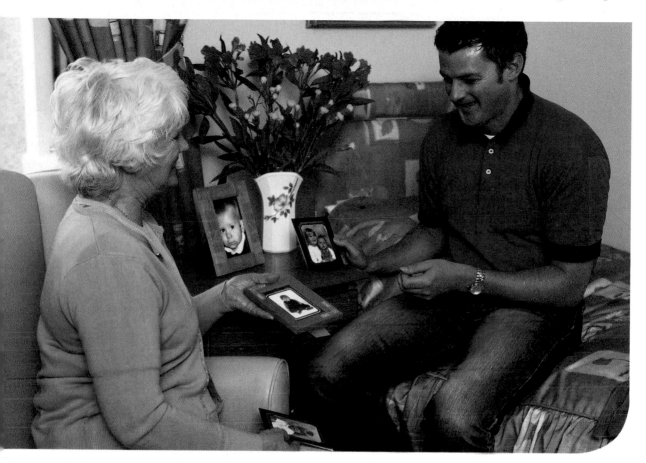

the emotional effect of the change on the person with dementia and on you. Talk to the staff at the home about how to manage the move.

The person may find it easier to settle in if there are familiar things in her room, such as some of her own furniture and ornaments. If possible, involve her – help her to choose what she would like to take.

Leaving the person for the first time on the day she moves in is likely to be difficult for both of you. Try to arrange things with the home so that there is something she can be involved in when you leave, such as a meal. And remember your own needs – is there someone who can be with you so that you don't have to go home alone?

Visits may also be emotionally difficult, especially at first. Some people with dementia settle in fast and are obviously happy in their new home, but others may not adjust so quickly. Some people find it better not to visit at first, to give the person a chance to settle in – ask the home staff for advice. Ask the home staff how she is when you are not there – perhaps the visits, while important, are a reminder for her of the change in her life. Give the person lots of reassurance. Remind yourself of the reasons why the decision was taken, and why this is the best choice for the person.

Most people find that the person settles in with time, and visiting gets more enjoyable. Your relationship may even improve now that you don't have to deal with day-to-day caring.

The home will put together a care plan for the person with dementia. You can give them important information about her needs and her likes and dislikes. If she has a life story book (see page 42) make sure she takes it to the home with her, so that staff can learn about her life. You can also say if you would like to be involved with her care; but don't feel that you 'ought' to do anything more than what you would like to do.

The booklet *Letting go without giving up: Continuing to care for the person with dementia,* available from the Dementia Helpline, is for carers who want to continue to be involved in the life of the person they have cared for. It looks at the impact of the move on the carer and on the person, and practical ways of staying involved and making visits more enjoyable.

If you are not satisfied with the care home

If you are not satisfied about the person's care at the home, you can make a complaint. All care homes must have a complaints policy. They should give you information about it if you ask.

First of all, speak or write to the person in charge of the home. If you are still not satisfied, you can talk to the social work department if they arranged the place in the home. Or you can contact the Care Commission (see **Further information,** page 103).

Loss and bereavement

at a glance

- Carers often feel loss throughout dementia.
- A move into long-stay care can cause a great sense of loss.
- When the person dies you may have a mixture of feelings; this is perfectly normal.
- Make sure you get support for yourself, and give yourself time.

Some carers say that dementia itself is like a long slow bereavement. You may feel that you are gradually losing the person you once knew. Many carers feel a great sense of loss when the person is admitted to long-stay care. Even when it is obvious that the person needs to move, some carers feel guilty at handing over much of the task of caring. Getting used to not being responsible for day-to-day caring can be hard. It may leave a big gap in your life. Talking about this with other carers can help, for example at a carers' support group. Even if you haven't been to a support group before, now might be a good time to join one.

Everyone is different and each person reacts to bereavement differently. Because of the 'slow bereavement' of dementia, many people find that their sorrow when the person dies is mixed with relief that so much suffering is over. Some people feel less sad than they feel they 'should', because they have already done so much grieving. Other feelings are common after a bereavement too, such as sadness, confusion, disbelief, anger or guilt. These mixed feelings are quite normal.

It takes time, of course, to come to terms with bereavement. At first most of your memories of the person with dementia may be about the years of the illness. This is when you may appreciate the help of family and old friends. Keep in touch with other carers too. They can help you come to terms with your feelings. Cruse Bereavement Care can help with bereavement counselling – see **Further information** on page 103.

You may find that feelings of stress and emotional upset stay for quite some time. But in time you will begin to remember the person before the illness. And eventually you will begin to pick up the threads of your own life again.

> *When my mother died after ten years of Alzheimer's disease, she was very different from her real self. In a way I felt I started to lose her long before she actually passed on. But she still left a huge gap in my life. It's now two years since her death, and I have managed to pick up the pieces of my own life again. Even though I will always miss her, the worst feelings are past now and I find I can remember her as she used to be before she got ill.*

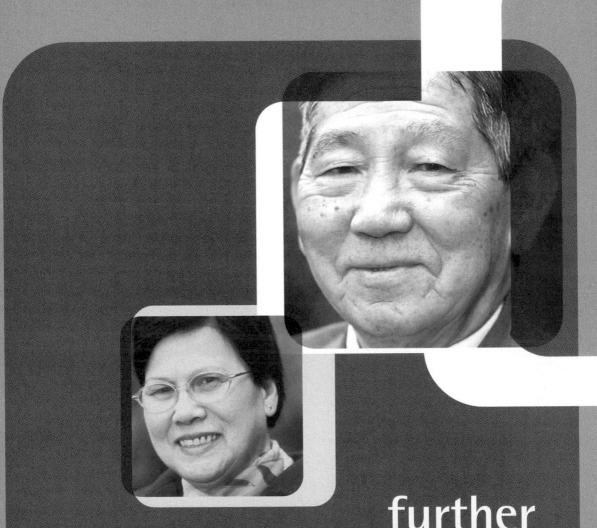

further information

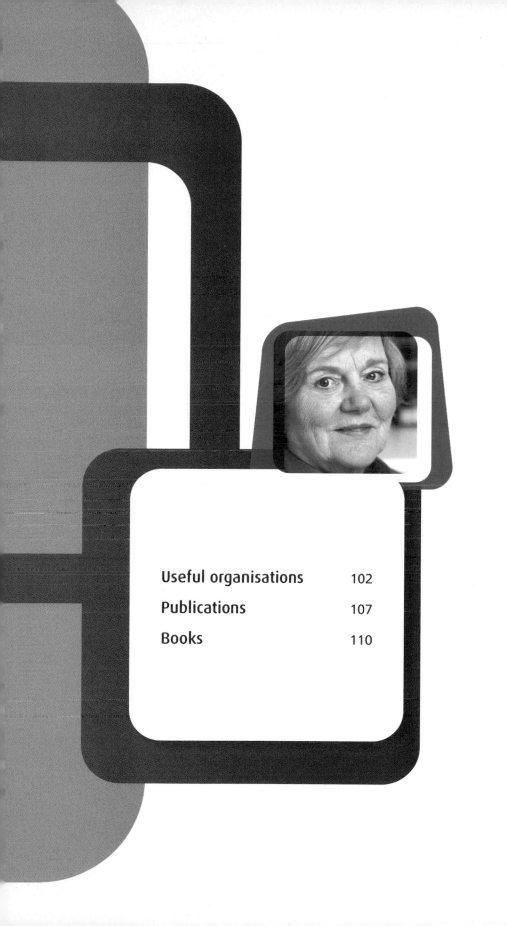

further information

Useful organisations

Age Concern Scotland

*Causewayside House, 160
Causewayside, Edinburgh EH9 1PR*

Office: 0845 833 0200; Age Concern
Information Line: 0800 00 99 66

Scottish Helpline for Older People:
0845 125 9732, textphone 0845 226
5851, open 10am – 4pm Monday to
Friday, calls charged at local rates

Web: www.ageconcernscotland.org.uk
email: enquiries@acscot.org.uk

Aims to improve the quality of life for
older people in Scotland. Supports a
network of over 400 local groups and
organisations. Provides advice and
information to all concerned with older
people. Factsheets available online or
from information line or send stamped
addressed envelope for publications list.

The Scottish Helpline for Older People
helps older people and those who
care for or work with older people.
Provides confidential information about
community care, tax, pensions, benefits
and other issues or puts callers in touch
with other services which can help.

Alzheimer Scotland

22 Drumsheugh Gardens, Edinburgh EH3 7RN

Office: 0131 243 1453; 24-hour Dementia
Helpline: 0808 808 3000 (freephone)

Web: www.alzscot.org
email: alzheimer@alzscot.org

Helps people with dementia, their carers and
families. Aims to be the national voice of
people with dementia and their carers and
works to improve public policies. Publishes
reports, information leaflets and booklets.
Provides services around Scotland, including
information, day care, home support,
befriending, courses for carers, carers' support
groups and the national 24-hour Dementia
Helpline. See website for wide range of
information and call the Dementia Helpline for
a free information pack or a publications list.

Alzheimer's Society

*Devon House, 58 St Katherine's Way,
London E1W 1JX*

Helpline: 0845 300 0336, open 8.30am
– 6.30pm Monday to Friday, calls charged
at local rates; office: 020 7423 3500

Web: www.alzheimers.org.uk
email: enquiries@alzheimers.org.uk

Helps people with dementia and their carers
and families in England, Wales and Northern
Ireland. Provides information and publications
and works to improve public policy. Local
branches provide services such as day care
and home support. Ask for a publications list.

Care Commission

Headquarters, Compass House, 11 Riverside Drive, Dundee DD1 4NY

Office: 01382 207100 or lo-call: 0845 60 30 890

Web: www.carecommission.com

The Care Commission regulates care services and oversees standards of care. It registers all care services in Scotland, including care homes and support services. Contact headquarters for details of your local Care Commission office, which can supply lists of care homes and support services in your area and copies of inspection reports.

Carers Scotland

91 Mitchell Street, Glasgow G1 3LN

CarersLine: 0808 808 7777 open Wednesday and Thursday, 10am – 12noon and 2pm – 4pm (freephone) office: 0141 221 9141

Web: www.carerscotland.org email: info@carerscotland.org

Campaigns and lobbies on behalf of all carers. Provides an information and advice service for carers and those interested in carers' issues. In addition to a direct information service, provides consultancy and support to a wide variety of carers' initiatives across Scotland and a training service on issues affecting carers including benefits, community care law, legislation and carer's assessments to workers in the statutory and voluntary sector.

Citizens Advice Bureau

See your phonebook for your local CAB or call Citizens Advice Scotland on 0131 550 1000

Web: www.cas.org.uk email: info@cas.org.uk

For advice and help with filling in forms for welfare benefits.

Crossroads Caring Scotland

Scottish Headquarters, 24 George Square, Glasgow G2 1EG

Tel: 0141 226 3793

Web: www.crossroads-scotland.co.uk email: info@crossroads-scotland.co.uk

Crossroads schemes across Scotland provide trained care attendants for home respite care.

Cruse Bereavement Care Scotland

Riverview House, Friarton Road, Perth PH2 8DF

Office: 01738 444 178 Fax: 01738 444 807

Web: www.crusescotland.org.uk email: info@crusescotland.org.uk

Provides free one-to-one bereavement counselling throughout Scotland. Call for details of local branches and publications.

Dementia Helpline

0808 808 3000 (freephone), 24 hours

Trained volunteers provide confidential information and emotional support to carers, people with dementia and their families and friends. Information is available on any subject to do with dementia, from where to find help to legal and financial matters. Run by Alzheimer Scotland.

Dementia Services Development Centre

Iris Murdoch Building, University of Stirling, Stirling FK9 4LA

Tel: 01786 467740

Web: www.dementia.stir.ac.uk
email: dementia@stir.ac.uk

Exists to extend and improve services for people with dementia and their carers. Provides information, development assistance, publications, website, research, training, conferences and seminars for managers, planners and providers of services in the statutory, voluntary and private sectors. Ask for a publications list or a training events brochure.

Department for Work and Pensions

Benefit Enquiry Line for People with Disabilities: 0800 88 22 00 or, for textphone users only, 0800 24 33 55. 8.30am – 6.30pm, Monday to Friday and 9am – 1pm on Saturday. Calls are free except from certain mobile phone networks. Help with applying for attendance allowance, disability allowance and carer's allowance.

Attendance Allowance and Disability Living Allowance Helpline: 0845 712 3456 – advice on existing claims.

Carer's Allowance: 01253 856 123

Pension Service: 0845 60 60 265 Monday to Friday 8am – 8pm – for benefits for people 60 and over.

Job Centre Plus: for benefits for people under 60 – see your local phonebook.

Web: www.dwp.gov.uk/
lifeevent/benefits/index.asp

Help the Aged Seniorline

0808 800 6565 (freephone). Lines open 9am – 4pm Monday to Friday

Information and advice for senior citizens, their relatives, carers and friends. Information available on welfare benefits, housing, health services, support for carers, care in the community, care homes, equipment and adaptations, insurance and sources of local help.

Legal Services Agency

Strathclyde and Lothian Mental Health Legal Representation Projects

3rd Floor, Fleming House, 134 Renfrew Street, Glasgow G3 6ST

Tel: 0141 353 3354

Web: www.lsa.org.uk
email: lsa@btconnect.com

and *Princes House, 3rd Floor, Rooms T9 & T11, 5 Shandwick Place, Edinburgh EH2 4RG*

Tel: 0131 228 9993

Web: www.lsa.org.uk
email: lsaedin@lsa.org.uk

Qualified solicitors give free and confidential advice on all aspects of the law relating to dementia. Legal representation is also available; there may be a charge for this, but you or the person with dementia may be able to get Legal Aid.

NHS 24

08454 24 24 24, calls charged at local rates; 24 hours

Web: www.nhs24.com

For health advice and support; part of NHS Scotland.

Pet Fostering Service Scotland

PO Box 6, Callander FK17 8ZU

Fostering requests: 01877 331496

Web: www.pfss.org.uk
email: info@pfss.org.uk

Organises volunteers to care for pets in an emergency. Scotland-wide – call for details of your local organiser.

Princess Royal Trust for Carers

Charles Oakley House, 125 West Regent Street, Glasgow G2 2SD

Tel: 0141 221 5066

Web: www.carers.org
email: infoscotland@carers.org

Provides information, support and practical help for carers. Supports a network of carers' centres. Also has a range of grant schemes for carers, including an Educational Bursary Scheme, a Carers' Relief Fund for carers in particular financial difficulties and a Young Carers' Fund.

Public Guardian

Office of the Public Guardian, Hadrian House, Callendar Business Park, Callendar Road, Falkirk FK1 1XR

Office: 01324 678300
Fax: 01324 678301

Web: www.publicguardian-scotland.gov.uk
email: opg@scotcourts.gov.uk

Call, write or see the website for forms and guidance. The Public Guardian registers continuing and welfare powers of attorney, authorisations to access funds, guardianship orders and intervention orders under the Adults with Incapacity Act. Supervises guardians and people granted an intervention order and will investigate any complaints about powers of attorney, accessing funds, guardianship or intervention orders, or any circumstances in which the property or financial affairs of an adult with incapacity appear to be at risk.

Scottish Government Health Directorates

Community Care Division, St Andrew's House, Regent Road, Edinburgh EH1 3DG

Web: www.show.scot.nhs.uk/sehd/ccd.asp

For community care guidance.

Scottish Government Justice Department

St Andrews House, Regent Road, Edinburgh EH1 3DG

Tel: 0131 244 2193
Fax: 0131 244 2195

Web: www.scotland.gov.uk/topics/justice/civil/awi
email: adultsincapacity@scotland.gsi.gov.uk

For Adults with Incapacity Act codes of practice and forms.

Scottish Independent Advocacy Alliance (SIAA)

Melrose House, 69a George Street, Edinburgh EH2 2JG

Office: 0131 260 5380

Web: www.siaa.org.uk
email: enquiry@siaa.org.uk

Have a directory of advocacy organisations and can help you to find advocacy locally.

Social Work Department

Look under the name of your local council in the phone book.

Deals with community care services, assessing the need for guardianship and other legal provisions. In some councils, it may be called something else, such as the Community Services Department.

Publications

Alzheimer Scotland booklets

All available in full text online at www.alzscot.org or free to carers in print or on tape from the Dementia Helpline on 0808 808 3000.

Activities: A guide for carers of people with dementia

For carers who look after someone who has moderate to severe dementia and need help with planning daily activities.

Dementia: Money and legal matters – a guide for carers

A comprehensive guide to planning for the future, benefits, community care rights and financial assessments.

Don't make the journey alone

Written by three people with dementia, this booklet offers personal thoughts, support and practical advice to people with a recent diagnosis.

Getting help from your doctor: A guide for people worried about their memory, people with dementia and carers

Looks at how dementia is diagnosed, treatments, getting help and support, keeping well and when the person with dementia should see the doctor again.

I'll get by with a little help from my friends: Information for friends of people with dementia

Written by carers, this booklet gives practical advice to help friends stay involved with both the person with dementia and the carer.

Letting go without giving up: Continuing to care for the person with dementia

For people who have been caring at home for a family member, partner or friend who is going into a care home. Aims to help carers establish new caring roles for themselves through visiting and through working as partners with care home staff.

Looking after yourself

Produced with the help of carers in Scotland, this booklet encourages carers to look after themselves as well as looking after the person with dementia.

A positive choice: Choosing long-stay care for a person with dementia

Based on the experiences of carers, this booklet gives practical information on long-stay care and help to deal with the emotional aspects. Includes information on help with care home fees and a checklist of what to look for when choosing a care home.

Talking dementia: A tape for carers (audio tape)

Explains dementia and looks at how to deal with problems, how to get help with caring and how to look after yourself as a carer. Includes interviews with carers and professionals.

Information sheets

Alzheimer Scotland also publishes a range of information sheets on topics including Alzheimer's disease, vascular dementia, Lewy body dementia, alcohol-related brain damage, drug treatments for dementia, travel and holidays, continence management, driving and dementia, when people with dementia walk and sexuality, plus local dementia service guides for many areas of Scotland.

Age Concern factsheets

Wide range of fact sheets available online at www.ageconcernscotland.org.uk or from the Age Concern Information Line on 0800 00 99 66 (ask for the Scottish versions). Titles include:

Factsheet 10 – Local authority charging procedures for care homes (including free personal care)

Factsheet 24 – Direct payments from social work

Factsheet 29 – Finding care home accommodation

Factsheet 38 – Treatment of the former home as capital for people in care homes

Factsheet 39 – Paying for care in a care home if you have a partner

Factsheet 40 – Transfer of assets and paying for care in a care home

Health Scotland booklets

Available free to carers from the Dementia Helpline and local health promotion departments.

Are you worried about your memory?

This booklet looks at what can cause forgetfulness and when to see the doctor if you are worried.

Facing dementia: Useful information for people with dementia

Information for people with early dementia and their carers, looking at practical arrangements and coping with feelings.

Keeping safe: A guide to safety when someone with dementia lives alone

Also useful for carers of people with dementia who do not live alone, this booklet looks at how to assess what is a risk, balancing risks and independence for people with dementia and practical steps you can take to help someone be safer.

Understanding dementia: A guide for young carers

A colourful booklet for 12 to 18-year-olds who are close to someone who has dementia. It explains dementia and looks at how to cope with its effects, encouraging young carers to look after themselves and to blame the illness, not the person with dementia or themselves.

Scottish Government Guidance

Guardianship and intervention orders - Making an application: a guide for carers

Available on the Scottish Government website at www.scotland.gov.uk/publications or free from:

Blackwell's Bookshop, 53 South Bridge Street, Edinburgh EH1 1YS

Tel: 0131 622 8283

Books

There are many books about dementia and about caring. This is just a small selection. Bookshops and libraries should be able to get these for you.

Books about caring and dementia

The 36 hour day: A family guide to caring for persons with Alzheimer's Disease, related dementing illnesses and memory loss in later life by Nancy L Mace and Peter V Rabins, Johns Hopkins University Press, ISBN 0801861497

Aimed at carers, this is a useful and clearly written book from the US, which covers most aspects of caring.

Caring for someone at a distance by Julie Spencer-Cingoz, Age Concern England, ISBN 0862423678

Examines what caring at a distance involves in practical and emotional terms.

Dementia – Alzheimer's and other dementias by Harry Cayton, Nori Graham, James Warner, Class Publishing, ISBN 1859590756

A handbook of information on dementia, in an easy to understand format. It covers diagnosis and treatment and practical, day-to-day problems.

Dementia reconsidered – the person comes first (rethinking ageing) by Tom Kitwood, Open University Press, ISBN 0335198554

A readable book, which reappraises older ideas about dementia, emphasises the personhood of men and women who have dementia and looks at a different approach to dementia care.

Understanding Dementia by Alan Jacques and Graham A Jackson, Churchill Livingstone, ISBN 0443055122

Explains dementia clearly and simply. Suitable for both carers and professionals who want to know more about the different causes of dementia and ways of coping with the problems the illness brings.

Understanding dementia: The man with the worried eyes by Richard Cheston and Michael Bender, Jessica Kingsley, ISBN 1853024791

Takes a person-centred approach to dementia, focusing on the importance of the experience and emotions of the person with dementia. Brings together ideas in dementia from social and clinical psychology, psychotherapy and linguistics.

Books by carers and people with dementia

In memory of memories: Experiences of living with dementia, Alzheimer's Society, ISBN 1872874681

A collection of writings first published in the Alzheimer's Society's newsletter by carers and two people with dementia.

Iris: A memoir of Iris Murdoch by John Bayley, Abacus, ISBN 0349112150

The writer Iris Murdoch developed Alzheimer's disease. This is a moving account by her husband of their life together and their experience of dealing with the illness.

Living in the labyrinth: A personal journey through the maze of Alzheimer's by Diana Friel McGowin, Delta, ISBN 0385313187

The author of this brave and powerful book was diagnosed with early-onset Alzheimer's disease in 1991.

Remind me who I am, again by Linda Grant, Granta Books, ISBN 1862072442

In 1993 the author's mother was diagnosed with multi-infarct dementia. This is an account of the illness and looks at the profound questions of identity, memory and autonomy that dementia raises.

The story of my father by Sue Miller, Bloomsbury, ISBN 0747565198

Sue Miller, an American author, cared for her father who had Alzheimer's disease. She recounts their lives, and the struggle to be fully with her father in his illness whilst dealing with her own fear of abandonment.